WHEN THE SOCCER BALL GOES FLAT

FABIENNE GAREAU RUDOLPH

ISBN 979-8-89112-733-3 (Paperback)
ISBN 979-8-89112-734-0 (Digital)

Covenant Books
11661 Hwy 707
Murrells Inlet, SC 29576
www.covenantbooks.com

To God, my Lord and Savior! I pray that this book will help and encourage you, the reader, and bless you beyond what you ask for.

THIS IS MY TRUE STORY AS BEST as I can remember it, frequently using personal journals, emails, texts, and my medical charts. They have helped me with the time frame such as dates and years of occurrences. Nevertheless, I've attempted to recall the memories and the feelings of those events; at no time were all the conversations meant to represent word-for-word accuracy.

A few names have been changed to protect the privacy of the individuals involved.

Unless otherwise noted, all Scripture quotations were the New International Version taken from Bible App—Read & Study Daily, an app by Olive Tree, version 7.13.4, by Gospel Technologies.

Half of the profits of this book will go to Cry Freedom Missions (https://www.cryfreedommissions.com/). They help reach, rescue, and restore survivors of human trafficking.

CONTENTS

ACKNOWLEDGEMENTS

To Ashely Rudolph, thank you for patiently reading and editing my manuscript twice, and thank you for all your encouragements. You are a great friend!

To Nancy Goff, I appreciate the time you took to correct my manuscript.

To John, my husband, and Melissa and Tristan, my children, thank you for all your encouragement, belief, and support in me. I love you!

The Bugle

IT ALL STARTED SEPTEMBER 15, 2021, FIVE days before my fifty-third birthday, when my mother-in-law called me.

"You wouldn't believe what happened to me!"

"What?" I responded.

"Yesterday, when I saw Annie Ruth, something happened! You know Annie Ruth is very religious, right? And something happened!"

Annie Ruth was a ninety-three-year-old neighbor who had recently lost her husband. She could barely walk and was shaking a lot, but she refused to leave her home. For that reason, members of her church would bring her meals and clean her house, and my mother-in-law would bring her mail every day.

I asked her, "What happened?"

"I don't want to tell you over the phone," she responded. "I will tell you on Wednesday when I bring your bowl of fruit for your birthday for when you go to the beach this weekend."

Wednesday afternoon, I watched my mother-in-law pull into my driveway, get out of her car, and carry a big bowl of fruit toward my house. I watched in awe at her resolve and strength. She had also lost her husband two years before and lived by herself. I admired her strength and courage as she carried the big bowl of fruit up my front steps. I took the bowl from her and put it in my fridge, and we both went to my den to talk about our week.

Finally, I asked, "What happened when you visited Annie Ruth?"

"I don't know, you will think I'm crazy—I haven't told anyone. It's not something you discuss. People will think I'm crazy! Promise you won't laugh."

"Tell me what happened, I will listen, and I won't laugh."

"I heard a bugle!" she said.

"A what?" I asked.

And my mother-in-law's story was the beginning of a new chapter in my life! She began to tell me all about her experience:

"When I delivered her mail that morning, she invited me in, and we sat at the kitchen table, talking. All of a sudden, I heard a bugle, like a trumpet but not a trumpet, a very loud noise like it was coming out of the walls. It scared me!" she narrated to me while also watching my reaction.

She kept on as she described the conversation they had:

"Annie Ruth, what was that loud noise? Was it an alarm?" she asked her.

Annie Ruth replied, "What did it sound like?"

"Like a loud trumpet but not a trumpet!"

"Oh! That's the bugle. God plays it every day for me. God is blessing you. I am so happy you heard it. Only one other person has heard it. You two are the only ones who have heard the bugle other than me!"

As my mother-in-law was speaking to me, I was wondering, *Could that be like the trumpet in the Bible?* Then I remembered it was called a shofar.

After she had left my house, I remembered that I could play the shofar on YouTube on my computer, and I called her right back.

"Okay, I will play it on my computer, and you should hear it on my speaker phone. Can you hear it?" I asked as I was playing the video.

She said, "That's it! That's what I heard, but it was not many different tones, just one blast, but that's it!"

Before we hung up, I casually mentioned that Annie Ruth would be such a neat person to meet.

The next afternoon, Peggy called me to tell me that Annie Ruth wanted to meet me, and we arranged to meet her the following Tuesday.

When Tuesday afternoon finally arrived, Peggy asked me if I wanted to walk over to her house, and when she saw me hesitating, she said, "It's okay. I will drive you because her driveway is very bumpy and full of branches and debris. It would be easy for you to fall!"

Dealing with my MS never gets any easier as I was thinking, *If an eighty-three-year-old woman can walk over there, so can I!* But I swallowed my pride and agreed to let her drive.

Once we arrived there, Peggy called her with her cell phone to open the garage door. I stretched my legs while we waited so I could walk better. When the garage opened, I saw her shaking with her walker and smiling a most beautiful smile, and she said, "I am so glad you came. I have been looking forward to it all week!"

When we sat down at her kitchen table, she said, "Please play the bugle!"

"What?"

I listened intently as she responded with slurred speech, "Please play the bugle!"

I opened my phone and played the shofar on YouTube. She smiled her most beautiful smile.

"That's it but with an even tone."

"That's the shofar. It is what they used in biblical times, I think."

She made me write it down so she could discuss it with her son. She proceeded to tell us how she hears the shofar every day and how Peggy and her friend heard it also.

"I hope you will hear it also while you're here and be blessed."

"That would be nice," I responded.

After telling us her life experiences with God, how he talks to her every day and how God wants her to live to tell others about him, she looked at me with piercing, brown eyes.

"Tell me about yourself!"

I was hesitating, and I wondered, *What do I tell this amazing woman of God, who has seen angels and hears from God?*

"Like what? My testimony?" I blurted out nervously.

"Yes, that would be great!" she said, smiling.

When I was done telling my story, I was very emotional, and she was too.

My mother-in-law later told me, "I have never heard you talk that long before!"

Afterward, I remember being so spent and exhausted and looking at the clock. We had been there two hours already. I was hot, and everything was a blur. I couldn't remember specifically her stories or the Bible passages that she kept mentioning. I just knew that I could feel the Holy Spirit in the room in a powerful way and that it was an amazing two hours.

As we were getting fidgety and thinking of leaving, Annie Ruth said, "Before you leave, I want you to learn a Bible quote and say it over and over. It will help with your MS."

"Fab…Fab," I heard and looked at her with a look of confusion because I didn't understand what she was saying, and Fab was definitely not in the Bible. So she decided to get up to get her Bible, and Peggy rushed to get the Bible for her.

"Give it to Fab! Now open it to 1 Peter 2:24, and where it says 'we' or 'you,' replace it with 'Fab,'" she instructed.

I read out loud, "'Who his own self bare *Fab's* sins in his own body on the tree, that *Fab*, being dead to sins, should live unto righteousness: by whose stripes *Fab* were healed.'

"Oh! Now I understand!"

And I read it again and wrote it down. I did not understand when she first told me because it was the old English from the King James version. When we were leaving, she was telling me again, "Every day, read that quote and learn it and say it 'til it becomes part of you."

When I got home, I opened my Bible app, the NIV version, on my phone and wrote 1 Peter 2:24 on a piece of paper by replacing "our sins" with "my sins" and so on:

"He himself bore my sins in his body on the cross, so that I might die to sins and live for righteousness; by his wounds I have been healed."

Then it became "Jesus, you yourself bore my sins with your body on the cross, so that I might die to sins and live for righteousness [your righteousness, not my righteousness]; by your stripes, your wounds, your suffering I have been healed."

I also highlighted it on my phone and, all week, repeated it throughout the day every day. However, I did not spend much time reading my Bible or studying the meaning of the Bible passage because I was so excited to see my improvement with my disease. The physical therapy I had started was allowing me to walk without my poles, and my balance was improving.

Every day, I did my stretching exercises and walking from 6 to 9 in the morning while listening to Christian music. The rest of the day, I worked and then fixed supper, and every twenty minutes or so, I would walk or stretch. At night, I walked again outside. I was following the instructions from my new physical therapist, and I was very excited with my improvement.

On Monday, October 19, like a student who has a big exam the next day, I decided to cram and prepare for my meeting with Annie Ruth the next day. My idea of preparing without cutting into my walking program was to listen to YouTube. I listened to several short videos explaining 1 Peter 2:24 while I stretched and walked outside. I invited the Holy Spirit to guide me and give me understanding.

To my surprise, this video made me angry, and I turned it off.

"God, I disagree with that!"

The video said that this scripture was not describing physical healing but spiritual healing and healing from my sins.

"God, why did you put Annie Ruth in my life and why did she say that this scripture would help my MS?"

And then I remembered another scripture, Mark 2:8–11:

> Immediately Jesus knew in his spirit that this was what they were thinking in their hearts, and he said to them, "Why are you thinking these things? Which is easier: to say to this paralyzed man, 'your sins are forgiven', or to say, 'Get up, take up your mat and walk'? But I want you to

know that the Son of Man has authority on earth to forgive sins." So he said to the man, "I tell you, get up, take your mat and go home."

And I prayed, "God, didn't you say 'Which is easier to say? Your sins are forgiven or get up and walk'? So, Lord, I claim your word! You forgive my sins, and you have healed me with your body on the cross."

I decided to listen to one more video and sat on the grass to do more stretches. It was a beautiful night, still warm, and the numerous stars were shining brightly. The video started, and I realized it wasn't about 1 Peter 2:24 at all; it was about Samuel, the prophet. I decided to listen to it and then go back inside. The video was about 1 Samuel 3:4–11, which states:

> …Then the LORD called Samuel.
>
> Samuel answered, "Here I am." And he ran to Eli and said, "Here I am; you called me."
>
> But Eli said, "I did not call; go back and lie down." So he went and lay down.
>
> Again the LORD called, "Samuel!" And Samuel got up and went to Eli and said, "Here I am; you called me."
>
> "My son," Eli said, "I did not call; go back and lie down."
>
> Now Samuel did not yet know the LORD: The word of the LORD had not yet been revealed to him.
>
> A third time the LORD called, "Samuel!" And Samuel got up and went to Eli and said, "Here I am; you called me."
>
> Then Eli realized that the LORD was calling the boy. So Eli told Samuel, "Go and lie down, and if he calls you, say, 'Speak, LORD, for your servant is listening.'" So Samuel went and lay down in his place.

> The LORD came and stood there, calling as
> at the other times, "Samuel! Samuel!"
> Then Samuel said, "Speak, for your servant
> is listening."
> And the LORD said to Samuel: "See, I am
> about to do something in Israel that will make
> the ears of everyone who hears about it tingle."

When the video was over, I prayed a simple prayer: "God, if you want to speak to me, use Annie Ruth to speak to me tomorrow, and I will listen," and then I went back inside the house.

When we arrived at Annie Ruth's house the next afternoon, I invited the Holy Spirit to be part of our meeting, got out of the car, and felt the warm sun. It was a beautiful autumn day that reminded me of a Canadian summer. I wanted to sit by the lake and just enjoy the fresh air.

As the garage door opened up, it brought me back to reality, and again, I saw her beautiful smile as she stood by the door with her walker. After a few pleasantries, we sat at the kitchen table, and right away, Annie Ruth looked at me and said, "God spoke to me this morning. He gave me a word for you! He wants you to write a book about your testimony. You have a beautiful testimony!"

She could have slapped me in the face! I was thinking, *"Oh my god, are you speaking to me? Oh! I asked you to talk to me! Oh! I can't write. I'm not a good writer!"*

She interrupted my thoughts. "Have you ever thought of writing a book with your testimony? You have a great testimony!"

At the time, I was so overwhelmed, and I would have liked to go home and think this through for myself, but I said, "I always felt like I should share my testimony, but I don't like public speaking, but I always told myself that if someone asked me, I would do it. But write a book—that's crazy!" I told her. "I am not good at writing at all! Good in math, but not writing."

Annie Ruth replied, "You should pray about it! God spoke to me that you should write a book. Pray about it."

"Okay, I will!" Then I added, "Last night, I was listening to a YouTube video, you know, the story when God talks to Samuel and he says, 'Here I am. Your servant is listening.' You know the story I'm talking about with Samuel and Eli who tells him it's God speaking to him?"

"Yes, I know that one!"

"Well, after watching the video, I prayed 'God, if you want to speak to me, use Annie Ruth to speak to me tomorrow!'"

Her eyes became moist, and she was very emotional. "God spoke to you, and he spoke to me—you need to pray to see if you should write the book."

"I will pray!" And as I said that, I knew I was going to write the book; it was clear as day to me that I was supposed to write the book. I was at peace with it! How was I going to do that? I had no idea! God was going to have to help me with this one!

Afterward, I asked Annie Ruth to repeat her stories to me, but again my mind kept wandering off, and I do not remember all the details.

When we were leaving, she said, "Remember, I want my son to pray for you!"

She called him and put him on the speakerphone.

Once again, I was put on the spot.

"What do you want me to pray for you?" her son asked.

I just blurted out "My walking! That my walking would be better, normal!"

He said, "Physical or spiritual?"

What is it with people—do they not think that God wants me to walk normal?

"Both!" I responded, "Both physical and spiritual! Oh yeah! Also, about the book!"

I was very thankful that they were praying for me, but once again, I was drained emotionally and physically, and I was zoning out and thinking about my book.

I went home, fixed a coffee, and then crashed on the couch! My husband walked in and asked, "How was Annie Ruth's?"

I described to him how the night before, I had listened to the Eli and Samuel story and how I had said a simple prayer to God to use Annie Ruth to speak to me and also how God spoke to Annie Ruth about me writing a book about my testimony!

I was curious to see how he was going to react and if he thought I was crazy.

He joked, "Great! We are going to be rich!"

And when my son Tristan walked in and John told him that I was going to write my story, he joked, "Great! We are going to be famous!"

We all laughed and enjoyed our time together! But I told them that if I write a book, it would be for God's glory, not my own!

To my surprise, John looked at me and said, "Seriously, Fab, I think that you should write a book and that you would be good at it. You will only have to make sure to have me read it and correct it and maybe also Aunt Nancy!"

If I felt at peace about it before, I certainly knew now, without a doubt, that with God's help and my husband's support, I was writing this book!

Part 1

Living the Dream

Go Home or Go Broke

Monday morning, September 7, 1987, my eyes slowly opened and were slow to focus. I looked around and noticed plain white walls.

Where am I? I wondered.

As I started to shift my legs around, I mumbled, "Ouch! *What the heck?*"

My quads, my hamstrings, and my calves were so sore that I could barely move, and then I remembered! I was lying in bed in my new dorm room at Sullivan Hall at NC State University, and I smiled!

Is this for real?

The soreness and the heaviness of my limbs were a true reality check, and I smiled again. I could hear my suitemates laughing in the bathroom that we all shared. Charmaine who had come with me from Canada and Michelle and Dione from Virginia, all freshmen, were recruited soccer players, ready to have a great time playing soccer for one of the best soccer teams in the NCAA and ready to enjoy the social life. I, on the other hand, was a walk-on!

Social life? That is not important right now!

And I started to worry as thoughts came flooding back in my mind:

Previously, two weeks ago, Coach Gross was driving us from Raleigh-Durham Airport to our dorm. If I wasn't so preoccupied, I would have noticed a city that was smaller than Ottawa, the capital of Canada, with no high-rises and less traffic! However, I just blurted out, "Coach, if I don't earn a full scholarship by next semester, I have to go back home! My dad had to borrow the money from his uncle for me to come here, and he said I only have one semester to play! So if you don't give me a full scholarship by next semester, I'm going home after this season!"

His response was not encouraging! "I will be honest with you! We already have three strikers who are very good and who have scholarships, and you probably won't be starting! I have no scholarships left that are available to give you!"

That comment could have destroyed me, but I remembered: *If Charmaine can get a scholarship, I can get one also,* but my stomach was in a big knot, and I didn't really feel brave at the moment!

The following day, Coach Gross asked two seniors, Barb Wickstrand, a goalie, and Amy Gray, a defender, to take us out to have a quick lunch at a fast-food restaurant. The purpose was for us to meet some of the experienced girls on the team, older girls, to answer all our questions and to make us feel welcomed.

At one point, Amy, always one to speak her mind, looked at me and said, "Coach Gross saw Charmaine play, and we know how good she is, but we don't know anything about you! Do you know a Canadian striker, Carrie Serwetnyk, who plays for Canada also? She also plays for UNC. That's a university down the road."

Charmaine responded, "Yeah! We know her. She also played with us on the Ontario team, with me and Fab!"

Amy looked at me again. "She's good, and she's very fast! Are you as good?"

"I'm better than her!"

"Are you as fast?"

"I'm faster!" I regretted blurting that out. I was so nervous, and I was thinking that *I was just being honest, but I don't think that came out the right way!* I just wanted to get back to my dorm room and get ready to play soccer. I really felt uncomfortable socially, and I was more comfortable on the field playing!

The next day, we had training camp or preseason, as it was called. We had two or three practices a day that went by like a blur. I didn't worry about making friends or socializing. Every single second that I was on the field, I didn't even think that the other girls were my teammates. I went as hard as I could, tackled hard, and bruised a few players, ran, and sprinted everywhere. I even slapped the ball out of Barb's hand—I was trying to get the goalie angry and off her game so I could score more goals in preseason. I didn't care what they thought because Coach Gross had made it clear: I was not starting and probably going home after this semester! For that reason, I was going down, knowing I had done my best!

Finally, Saturday came, September 5, 1987[1]. It was a beautiful, hot, sunny day; we were sitting in the meeting room near our locker room, waiting for Coach Gross to give us the starting lineup for the first game of the season. He was telling us that playing Central Florida was the big game. We were ranked seventh nationally, and they were ranked ninth. This was the most important game of the weekend because it would affect the Southern Division Rankings at the end of the season.

"Lori Kerrigan, you will mark Michelle Akers. She's on the national team, and she's their best player!" he said[2].

When he was done, he started announcing the starting lineup, which I thought didn't affect me. He had been clear about that. I remembered correctly; now I just had to perform if I went in as a sub.

As I was pondering this, I heard loud and clear: "Charmaine at center forward and Debbie and Fab on the wings up front!"

That's me! That's me! I'm starting!

I was so excited but so nervous!

Looking back, I am so amazed at what an incredible weekend it was for me! We were losing, 1–0, against Central Florida when Kerrigan tied the game up! Just like in a dream, I scored the winning goal in overtime in my first collegiate game! I didn't think life could get much better than that, but I scored two more goals the next day when we beat George Mason, 3–0![3]

After thinking about it, I was surely going to get the scholarship! I came as a freshman, a striker, and scored three goals in two games, and that's the job of a striker! And then my hopes began to sink again as I remembered he didn't have any scholarships available to give this year! My hopes deescalated even lower when I remembered that I had had almost the same experience less than a month ago!

Earlier that same summer, I was sitting on a bed in a dorm room except it was at St. John's-Ravenscourt, a university preparatory school in Winnipeg City, Canada![4] I was waiting impatiently for the list of players who had made the Women's Canadian National Team. I was also pondering while sitting on the bed how I had gotten there. It had been a long road but a fun one.

When I came back to Ottawa at fifteen, I had joined the Nepean Soccer Team in my age group because I was told that it was the best team in the Canadian capital for my age group. After my first game, I received a phone call from Stewart, the coach of the Women's Nepean Team.

"Hi, I'm Stewart, the coach of the Women's Senior Team, and I think you might want to move up to our team. The level of soccer would be much better for you! Anyways, in a couple days, we are having a scrimmage in a gym, and you should come and play to see if you would like it. I want you to play with this girl, Charmaine Hooper! I think you would love to play up front with her!"

Being one to never turn down a fun sport game of any kind, I showed up to the scrimmage. As always, I was super nervous and shy and scared to meet new people. You could say that there was nothing average about me! As much as I was extremely confident in any sport, I *was* very awkward socially! However, as soon as we started playing, I had the best time! Charmaine was good; she was great! It was the first time that I met a female athlete who was as good or better than me.

After the scrimmage, as we were sitting on the bleachers, I learned that, like me, she grew up having to play sports with boys or her brothers because girls were never good enough or interested! Back then, it was not a fad for all girls to work out or participate in sports like today!

As I was sitting on my bed in the dorm, reminiscing about the past few years, my thoughts kept being interrupted by the nervous chatter and laughter from Charmaine and several other girls waiting in the hallways of the Canadian school. My mind drifted away from their conversation back to my thoughts and to what Charmaine and I had gone through together to make it.

Most days that we had club practice, I would take the city bus to Charmaine's house, an hour ride, and hang out with her until practice. Other times, I would go directly to the field and work on my shots or dribbling until everyone got there. On weekends, we were playing games with the club or we would travel five hours on the Greyhound bus to train on the women's provincial team in the Toronto area, the biggest city in Canada.

Then, out of the blue, my mom announced to me, "Your dad and I can't afford to pay for your travels to Toronto anymore and support your high school sports and all your siblings' sports also."

This put me in a very difficult situation because I also loved playing all the high school sports; I played basketball, volleyball, badminton, and soccer for my high school at the time.

"Papa, I have to play for Ontario so I make the national team someday! I cannot stop now!" I begged him.

"How can you be on the national team when a women's national team doesn't exist?" he asked.

"One day, there will be a national team, so I have to keep playing on the Ontario team!"

"You have to be realistic—there is no team right now!" he repeated.

My answer to my situation and his comments was to stop going to school, get a day job cleaning houses for the elderly, which my mom had helped me get, and take my last high school course at night school. This allowed me to keep training with the provincial team while graduating from high school!

"Hey!" someone shouted, and my heart started beating a hundred miles per hour. "They posted the list!"

I was quickly brought back to reality at St. John's-Ravenscourt School, full of nervous soccer players.

I took a deep breath, slowly got off my bed, feeling all my aching muscles from playing so many intense games, and headed down the hall. We had just finished playing a tournament where all the provincial teams played one another, and the scouts watched us to select players who would leave the next day for national camp! Charmaine and I played striker for Ontario, and we had just won the whole tournament for the second year in a row! We were the Canadian champs, but that didn't matter to us! I rushed down the hallway; the only thing that did matter was thinking, *Is my name on the list?*

When I arrived to where the list was posted, it was surrounded by a bunch of girls. It was loud; there was laughter and crying, yelling and silence—no in between! It was also a very awkward moment. The ones who had made the team smiled but tried to control it so as not to hurt their teammates who were not as fortunate girls who had also sacrificed a lot, with a lot of hard work and sweat. I personally had even missed my prom night because the provincial team was practicing that same weekend!

As I pushed my way through the crowd, I noticed Charmaine avoiding looking at me, and instantly, I had a bad premonition! Finally, I walked to the area in front of the posted list as girls looked down at their feet and stepped sideways to let me through. With so many butterflies flying around in my stomach, I read the list! I didn't see my name, and I felt sick! I saw Charmaine's name! I read the list a second time, and again, I didn't see my name, and now my legs felt like they were going to buckle!

From that point on, everything was a blur: Charmaine talking to me, our coach saying that I had played well, the team meeting, and the selected girls departing with the national team to go play against the American team across the border in Blaine, Minnesota[5]. To make matters worse, the exact thing had happened to me the previous year! For the second year in a row, I had won the national championship with the Ontario team, but I was not selected for the national team!

In a state of shock and haze, I packed my bags, wished Charmaine good luck, and boarded the team van of "the unwanted" from Ontario!

Later, I held it together on the plane. In my head, thoughts were going around over and over. I did not understand because I had played well. In my mind, I was as good as Charmaine or close to it, and we had just won the nationals. Unlike the previous year, I had a good tournament; what else could I do? I had given everything I had! I do not recall much about the plane ride from Winnipeg to Toronto, but as if it was yesterday, I remember sitting in the back of the Greyhound bus on the way to Ottawa from Toronto and crying, tears rolling down my face—my dreams shattered! It was the sharpest pain I had ever felt in my young life!

After a five-hour bus ride in the back of the bus, crying and replaying all the training and hurdles leading up to the tournament and then replaying all the games of the tournament down to the miniscule details, like reruns of a good movie that you have watched a hundred times, I was resolute in my new plan not to go to university!

As I was stepping down from the bus in the Ottawa station parking lot, I spotted my mom sitting in her car, a blue Renault. Before she could get out of her car, I made a sign for her to wait, proceeded to where the bus driver was downloading the bags, and thanked him as I grabbed my bag. I walked toward the back of the car, and my mom, who couldn't help herself, came rushing out and hugged me! Instantly, the tears rolled down my face again, and I hurried inside on the passenger's side as my mom put the bags in the back of the car and joined me. My mom looked at me compassionately and said, "I am so sorry!" I wiped my eyes again and started venting my frustrations, words gushing out like Noah's flood!

After unloading all my frustrations, I looked at my mom and said, "Maman, I've decided not to go to university! Before you interrupt me, hear me out! I know it's important to you for me to go to school, but the best soccer is in Montreal, Quebec, and Vancouver, British Columbia—half the girls on the national team train in Vancouver with the national team coach and the other half in Montreal with the assistant coach. So I think I will go to Vancouver and get a job there until I make the team!"

"*But, Fabienne,* you have to go to university to get a good job! And you know how important it is for your dad also because he knows how hard it was for him with a grade 10 education to take courses in trade school! *Soccer will not get you a job!*"

Like a teenager or, more precisely, like a young adult who knows it all, I responded forcefully, "I've made up my mind! Maybe I can go later!"

My mom kept trying to convince me to no avail. My young mind was made up!

A couple weeks later, I was lying on my bed, feeling sorry for myself when I heard my mom yell "Fab, Charmaine is on the phone!"

I took a deep breath as I was thinking to tell her *I'm not here*, but curiosity won the battle in my head. I got up and ran out of the room and picked up the phone.

"Hi, Charmaine!"

"Hey, how are you? Sorry about you not making the team!"

I interrupted quickly, "How was camp? The game against the US?"

"Camp was great. I'm so sore! But we got hammered by the Americans! Our team sucks compared to them! We lost, 4–2, against the US[5]. And we also lost, 2–0, against Sweden."[6]

As she went on and on about camp and the games, my mind drifted again. The same movie started playing in my head about *why I did not make the team when I thought I was better than some of them! What now?*

Charmaine interrupted my thoughts. "Guess what?"

"What?" I said, struggling through this conversation.

"I got a full scholarship to go play in the US at NC State University. It's thirty minutes from the school, UNC, that we sent our recruiting tape to!"

Now she had my full attention!

"How did that happen?"

She proceeded to tell me that several coaches from American universities were scouting players during camp and the games. After the game against the US, Larry Gross, the head coach of NC State women's team, approached her and offered her a full ride, right there, just like that! And all those video tapes and letters that we had sent to several American universities and not one response! She had been filling out a bunch of paperwork to attend NCSU, and it was pretty much a done deal!

"Did you give him my name?" I asked bluntly.

Charmaine was aware that I also wanted to go play in the US after sending all those videos and letters!

"Yes, I did! But he said he had already given away all his scholarships for the year!"

"Can you please call him back and give him my name and phone number and tell him how I'm good enough and that I'm very interested in playing for him!"

"Sure! I can do that!"

"Thank you!"

Now I was so excited!

I'm not sure what Charmaine told him and what kind of sales pitch she used, but he called me within the hour! When I picked up the phone and said "hello," he proceeded in making his own sales pitch, and of course, I was easily sold! I told him that, yes, I was interested in playing for him and that was what I wanted more than anything else!

He said, "Great! Now let me talk to your dad or mom! We have to discuss the finances!"

I yelled as I handed her the phone, "Maman! The soccer coach from NC State University is on the phone! He wants to talk to you about me playing for him in the US! Charmaine is going also! Please say yes!"

After what seemed like an eternity, my mom got off the phone. Before she had a chance to say anything, I exclaimed, "Please let me go and pay for me to go!"

"Fabienne, I'm so sorry, but it's too much money for you to go. He said we have to show that we have over thirty thousand dollars in our bank account because you're a foreign student, and that's American money! With the exchange, one hundred US dollars is one hundred thirty Canadian dollars![7] We don't have that kind of money!"

"But Coach Gross said if I played well the first season, I could earn a full scholarship for the following year!" I pleaded.

"I'm sorry! Maybe you will hear back from one of those schools you sent your videos to!" Mom countered.

"I didn't hear back from any of them," I blurted out as I ran to my room and slammed the door. Similarly, when I didn't make the national team, I cried, feeling defeated once again!

Later, as I was eating dinner with my mom and my three siblings, my heart was not into it, and I didn't even notice that my dad was missing. As I was moving my food around with my fork and making different piles of food on my plate but not really eating, my dad walked in. With a big grin, he announced, "Fab! We have to talk! Let's go to your room!"

"Why?"

"Come on—you will be glad to hear this."

Reluctantly, I followed him to the bedroom and closed the door behind me.

"What?" I said with a big frown on my face that said "What the heck are we doing here!"

With the biggest grin I'd ever seen on my dad's face, he said, "You are going to North Carolina to play soccer!

"But how? Maman said that you didn't have enough money." I didn't want to get my hopes too high and be hurt once again!

I looked at my dad expectantly, and I realized that I had never seen my dad's face so radiant before. He was beaming with excitement when he started to explain to me that he went to see his rich uncle. To this day, I don't even know his name! He described to him that when he was seventeen, he had a chance to play hockey in the juniors, but his dad told him no because he was too small. My dad was a little shorter than five feet six with a small frame. He also explained to his uncle that he didn't want to take away my dream in the same way that it was taken away from him. He then asked his uncle if he could borrow about thirty thousand dollars to pay for one semester.

"Fab, that was the most difficult thing for me to do, but I want you to live your dream! You have six months to battle and win a full scholarship for next semester! Make sure you tell your coach that after the first semester, you are going back home because your parents have no more money! That's very important that as soon as you see him, tell him that you only have six months unless he gives you a full ride!"

I ran into his arms, and we held each other for a long moment, both of us with tears rolling down our faces!

"Merci, Papa!" I whispered in his ear.

What an amazing thing that my parents had just done for me—*what love*! They had just opened the door wide open for me to live out my dreams! I ran to the kitchen, with my dad close behind me, still smiling, and hugged my mom.

"Merci, Maman! I'm going to North Carolina State University to play soccer!"

"And study!" she reminded me as a good mom should.

I sat at the table and devoured my now cold food like a hungry wolf as the family discussed all the preparations that needed to be done.

After supper, I called Charmaine.

"Guess what? I'm going to NC with you! Thanks for talking to the coach for me!"

"Did he offer you a scholarship?"

"No! I'm going to be a walk-on! That's what he called it, and he explained that I will not have a scholarship and that it will be like a tryout for me. So my dad said that I have one semester to earn one. If not, I come back home! *One semester! Do or die!*"

I came back to my reality on that Monday in North Carolina when Charmaine walked back into the dorm room.

"Hey! Are you okay?"

"I'm fine! I'm just so sore from the two games we played this weekend, but that was so much fun."

"But is something bothering you?" she asked.

I was saved by the phone ringing, a landline (we didn't have any cell phones at that time). I picked up the phone.

"Hello!"

"Fab, it's Coach Gross! I need to see you right away! *It's urgent!* I want you to come to my office in Case," a building where the coaches had offices and athletes ate in the cafeteria.

"Is something wrong?"

"We can't discuss it over the phone! I want you to come and see me right away!"

"Okay, I will be right there!" I said with butterflies flying around in my stomach and legs still aching.

The ten-minute walk from my dorm to his office seemed like an eternity. I rushed into his office.

"Is something wrong?" *Am I going home early?*

"Sit down!"

I walked to the chair in front of his desk and sat down, looking expectantly at him.

He smiled and said, "I just want to tell you that you had a great training camp, so I decided to start you in both games, and then you scored three goals in two games. Well, the girl who was supposed to start in your place decided to go home!"

"Is she sick? Or is something wrong with her?" *Why did he call me to tell me that it was urgent?* I wondered.

"No! She quit our team and went home! She decided that it was not for her. I wanted to tell you that she had a full scholarship, and I've decided to give you her full ride!"

"Are you serious?"

"Yes! You have a full ride for four years! Do you want to call your dad and tell him yourself?"

I was trying to hold it together emotionally. Years of training and desiring to play sports at the highest level, I was so ecstatic! So much joy! "Yes!" I barely whispered, trying to hold it together! "Yes!" I said more loudly!

He pushed the phone toward me, and I dialed my parents' number. I don't remember why my dad was home, but he answered the phone.

"Allo!"

And I told him in French that I had a great camp, scored three goals in the first two games, then one striker quit and went home, and I got her full scholarship!

He yelled the same way the Hispanic TV announcers call a goal in a soccer game, "*Goallllllll!*" But he yelled "*Wooooooooo!*"

That was the best moment I had ever shared with my dad!

CHAPTER 2

Childhood Olympic Dream

Now, LOOKING BACK AT MY FRESHMEN YEAR at NC State, I did not cherish the moment I was living in nor realize how special it really was. Every day was so much fun, playing and training with some of the best players in the country! We became so close as a group practicing together, battling other teams, and getting to travel around the country playing soccer. We also became very good friends as we shared our studies and social life together!

At the time, I enjoyed playing sports so much that I didn't realize what I was really accomplishing as a walk-on freshman: fifth in ACC points, third in ACC goals, All-ACC Team, All-ACC Weekend Team[1], and All-American Freshman![2]

Moreover, I certainly did not know who Jim Valvano was when I attended the NC State Sports Banquet and received the Women's Soccer Best Offensive Player Award in front of a crowd of Wolfpack Athletes! I didn't know how spoiled we really were: getting free shoes, having someone washing our training clothes and uniforms, our own locker rooms, trainers on demand, and our own cafeteria, and the list goes on. Honestly, I would have been just as happy playing with the team in my backyard wearing rags! Sports were my life, and this was better than I could have imagined!

When my freshman season ended and when I thought that my life couldn't get more perfect, my phone began to ring. I picked up the phone and said, "Hello!"

"May I speak to Fabienne Gareau?" the stranger asked.

"Speaking!"

"This is Neil Turnbull, coach of the Canadian Women's National Team. After watching you with the Ontario Team last summer, I have been following your soccer freshman year at NC State. You had a great season, and I would like to invite you to the next training camp. After camp, we will select the thirty best players for the team!"

A month later, in December 1987, I attended training camp and made the Women's Canadian Soccer Team! *I was living my fairy tale!*

Presently, as I am mulling over my freshman year and that phone call, I vividly remember declaring my life destiny to my mom as an eight-year-old child:

"Hurry! Hurry! We need to go down the hill! I don't want to miss the Olympic torch! Can we go *now*?" I yelled as I ran through the house as a small bundle of energy.

"We're okay. We still have an hour and a half before they go by!" my mom responded in French.

I grew up in a French-Canadian home. At the time, I only spoke French and went to a French school and a French church, and everyone on my street also spoke French.

"I don't want to miss it! I'm going now, and you can join me later!" I said with animation.

"No! You will wait for me, and we won't miss the torch!"

On the afternoon of July 15, 1976, as I was pacing up and down, waiting in our home, located in Cumberland, Ontario, I pondered in amazement how far the Olympic torch had traveled for the Montreal Olympics! My mom had explained to me that the Olympic flame traveled in Greece from Olympia to Athens, and after that, she didn't completely understand, but from there, the flame was converted into impulses that were transmitted by satellite.[3]

Today, in Ottawa, a receiver picked up the signal and triggered a laser beam that recreated the flame, starting the Canadian leg of the torch's journey to Montreal. It was the first time such technology had been used to transmit the Olympic flame. The prime minister, Pierre Elliott Trudeau, had just given the starting signal to the first runners in the Ottawa-Montreal relay at 3:00 p.m[4].

My mom also explained to me that a group of twelve bearers from different regions had lighted more torches for the ceremonial one-kilometer run, and then again, it was combined in one flame as they passed it on to the runner who took over the relay for the second kilometer.

And now they were traveling between Ottawa and Montreal, along the Ottawa River, passing successively from one bank to the other[5]. *And that meant that they were on their way, and soon they would be on the road, down the hill!*

Earlier that year, my mom had also explained to me how they were recruiting torchbearers to run each kilometer from Ottawa to Montreal.

"I want to do it, Mom! I can run fast. I want to carry the torch!"

"No, you can't! The advertisement says that you have to be fifteen years old, and you're only eight!" my mom patiently explained to me. "Plus I heard that there are more than four thousand applicants for just over seven hundred positions, and you have to be able to run a kilometer in five minutes or less."[6]

"I can do that in five minutes. I will show you. We can go outside, and you can time me when I run it," I had said.

Again she explained that I had to be fifteen years old.

"That's not fair," I huffed as I stormed out the room.

Finally, forty-five minutes later, my mom said, "Okay, let's go down the hill."

We lived on Rue Gerald, a nice, quiet neighborhood with houses on each side of one road coming off old Highway 17, east of Ottawa, Ontario. At the time, it was a small town, only a twenty-minute drive east of Ottawa. For an active child as I was, it was a fun place to grow up! I had many friends with which to play hide-and-seek and numerous sports and games. At the end of the road, on the top of the hill, there were also some woods with numerous trails and a nice fall to explore and perfect for sledding in the winter.

As we were walking down the road, I saw numerous families and kids making their way down, and some of them were already assembled, waiting for the Olympic torch!

Marc yelled at me, "Fabie [my childhood nickname]! We're going to run with the person with the torch!"

"Yeah! That will be fun." I laughed.

"Wait! Just for a minute," my mom said as she and I joined the group of children and parents on both sides of the runner, waiting for the torch.

"Look! The flame is coming!" someone yelled.

The smiling runner ran toward the awaiting runner, who was surrounded by us, and slowed down, and they both joined their torches until the flame passed to the awaiting runner. I was speechless as I observed in awe! Then the new torchbearer held his torch and began his run followed by all of us! As I ran with the group, I could hear the rest of the spectators applauding and encouraging. To me, that was the most incredible feeling.

Shortly after, no longer able to keep up with the runner, we stopped and started walking back; I couldn't stop smiling. I looked at my mom and said, *Someday, I will be in the Olympics!* And I believed that with all my soul.

CHAPTER 3

Cloud Nine and Then Some More

MY FRESHMAN YEAR WAS JUST THE BEGINNING! After making the Canadian National Team, getting my surgery to remove bone spurs in my right foot, and training the rest of the summer to be super fit, I was excited to start my sophomore year!

In training camp, we met our new assistant coaches, Jerry and Jill Ellis. Jill had just finished her senior year at William & Mary and had also been an excellent forward. She asked me if she could train me before each practice, and I learned all the skills of a striker: how to turn when the defender is on your back and how to turn when you have a lot of space, how to shoot, etc.

As my skills improved, we added midfielders and defenders to our training so we could learn combination plays and how I could make diagonal runs behind defenders or learn when to pass back. *I loved it—I couldn't get enough!*

My sophomore year with our new assistant coaches was great! My 1988 women's soccer season is still considered the Wolfpack's best year in their history. The team finished with a 19–2–3 record[1]. We ended up winning the ACC's in penalty kicks against our archrival UNC! We met again in the NCAA finals, but they destroyed us, 4–1.

Looking back, I wish we could have switched those two games where they win the ACC's and we win the NCAA's. *My fairy tale was still rolling*—how many players can claim to be fortunate enough to have a personal coach like Jill Ellis, who ended up coaching the US women's soccer team and winning two World Cups. She is also the all-time leading American coach in wins with 106![2]

Afterward, I had to redshirt my junior year in 1989 because mono landed me in the hospital. My parents picked me up at the hospital and drove me back to Canada in my uncle's van where I could lie in the back for the fifteen-hour drive back home. I spent the whole fall semester at home, convalescing while missing soccer season and friends.

Amazingly, my most vivid memory occurred the following year in the fall of 1990 when I replayed my junior year of soccer. We were playing UNC, our nemesis, in the quarterfinals! It occurred at UNC on the beautiful pitch located inside the running track. I looked up while I was warming up and saw an ocean of people, all wearing sky-blue shirts, in the packed stadium seats, and I was so nervous yet excited to be there. I looked up to the opposing team, and there were Mia Hamm and Christine Lilly, considered the best two strikers in the world! Then I noticed Linda Hamilton, the best sweeper, who had just transferred from our team to their team, and I smiled. I was so motivated. We had Charmaine Hooper and me, both playing for NC State and Canada as strikers. I felt really good about our team! Just to name a few, Charmaine Hooper, Jill Rutten, Colette Cuningham, Kim Yankowsky, Lindsay Brecher, Meaghan Owins, and Mary Pitera. Some had made the American training camp, and some would end up playing professionally. However, if they were the same caliber as a UNC player, they all knew the UNC player would be chosen for the national team because the UNC coach was none other than Anson Dorrance, also the national team coach! We were all a motivated Wolfpack!

In the first half of the back-and-forth battles and attacks, UNC's Kristine Lilly first blasted a thirty-yard shot over Lindsay Brecher's head and hit the crossbar. Twenty-three minutes into the contest, NC State's Charmaine ripped a shot by goalkeeper Proost, only to be saved by defender Laura Boones's head. Eleven minutes later, NCSU midfielder Jill Rutten rifled a twenty-yard penalty shot that was saved by Proost off the post. Finally, with thirty-eight seconds left, the 0–0 tie was finally broken by UNC's Mia Hamm who finished off a cross on the twelve-yard line. It was shortly followed by a pack attack with Charmaine blasting a shot as I was sprinting toward the goal in case there was a rebound, the ball hitting the post, and then hearing the horn signaling the end of the half—*no rebounds for me! Bummer!*[3] It remained 1–0 as we walked to the locker rooms for our halftime break.

Fifteen seconds into the second half, NC State's Jodi Osborne dribbled down the right flank and crossed the ball; it was a driven ball, hard and low to the near post. I sprinted toward the near post and surprised my defender by getting the inside position. I dove forward and headed the ball into the goal.[4] All the Wolfpack players ran and yelled as we embraced! We felt euphoria! We knew we had this. All of us were thinking, *If we can beat UNC, we can win the NCAA's!*

The second half remained tied and was a bloodbath with many fouls. It was reported that fifty-eight fouls were committed in that brutal match and resulted in several minor injuries.[3] In the last fifteen minutes, Charmaine scored, but it was disallowed because of a foul committed. A few minutes later, after one of those fouls, I received a long ball, broke past two defenders, and dribbled around the goaltender Proost on the left side of the penalty area. Next thing I knew, I went flying up into the air when Proost took me out. A penalty shot was awarded to us, and Jill Rutten put the ball in the back of the net!ic[4]

To my horror, in the last five minutes of the second half, our coach decided to take Kim Yankowski out to give her a short rest. *What are you doing? What an idiot, she's marking Chris Lilly, and she hasn't done any damage*, I processed in my mind. Sure enough, UNC, with their backs against the wall, pushed everyone forward in the attack. NC State committed a foul just outside the box. Mia Hamm took the free kick and tapped the ball to Kristine Lilly who scored off a funny bounce. Again, we ended the half tied up, 2–2.[4]

As both sides were resting on the sidelines, the referees blew the whistle to get the first overtime half started. Shortly into the overtime, NCSU Collette dribbled past defenders to the top of the box and passed a square ball to Rutten who riffled the ball into the net. The score was 3–2, Wolfpack leading![4]

Like a replay of a horrible movie, our coach took out Kim Yankowski who was marking Chris Lilly, who, once again, scored and tied the game.[4] Finally, in the last two minutes of the second overtime, Mia Hamm took a corner on the right side, and Rita Tower headed it in our goal![5] We lost, 4–3, in double overtime, and that was so painful, so emotional, so raw. We had left everything on the field! To this day, that was the most exciting game I have ever participated in! At the time, *Soccer America*, a popular soccer newspaper, dubbed the game "The Greatest Game in Women's Soccer History."[6]

CHAPTER 4

Big Plans, Big Crash

AFTER THE WAY OUR SEASON HAD ENDED, I had big plans for my summer before the senior year. The big picture was to keep getting better and better. And why not? I aimed to be one of the best players in the world and attempt to win the NCAA with my teammates. I believed that with hard work and with my natural athletic ability, the sky was the limit. So many players I knew were playing professionally in Japan or Europe and getting paid. *Getting paid to play sports!* And then if that didn't pan out, I could go back to Canada and do everything I needed to do to play hockey for the Canadian Women's National Team. Canada always won the World Cup and ended up winning two gold medals in the Olympics in hockey.

My dad had just called me and said, "Fab, I just went to see the women's national team play hockey in Ottawa, and I think that you could play on that team."

Surprisedly, that comment made me angry inside, and after I hung up, it brought back this childhood memory:

"Papa, I want to play hockey on a team! Daniel plays, and he's only seven! I'm nine!" I moaned.

"You can't! Girls don't play hockey!" And no sooner than it came out of his mouth, he realized what a mistake it was to say that to his oldest child. She had always been a spunky, active girl who never stopped running, jumping, and climbing trees. He also knew too well not to tell her that she couldn't do something. In general, she was a good kid and never caused any problems. She was a very happy child. The exception to that rule was when she was told that she couldn't do something. For that reason, he quickly rephrased that. "I mean that right now. There are no girls' teams."

I quickly answered, "That's okay. I can play on a boys' team! You know that I play with the Maisonneuves and their friends almost every day, and those boys are four years older than I am. We play hockey at the neighborhood rink and in the basement all the time!"

As an adult, my dad had told me that I would come home after our neighborhood hockey games full of bruises and that it would bother him but that I just loved it! The boys, being older than me, a girl, would put me in goal and would start shooting harder and harder when they failed to score!

"I'm sorry, but I can't let you play! In Bantam hockey, ages thirteen to fourteen years old, they start playing body contact, and at that age, the boys get stronger than girls!"

"But I play with boys that age now!" I said angrily.

"I said no, and that's final! End of discussion!" My dad stood his ground.

I stormed out of the house, and I started running up the hill to the end of the road. I entered the woods, my sanctuary and my escape. It was hard to get privacy in our home, being the oldest of four children: Daniel, my brother; Julie, my sister; and Melanie, my sister who had just been born. Out of breath, I started walking down the trail that would lead me to the falls. Midway through the path, halfway down a hill, I just dropped to the ground and started sobbing.

How could he do that to me? That was what I really loved. How can I not play with boys in a league when I play with them every day? That is not fair, and Dan plays, and we have to go watch him all the time.

As my sobbing slowly subsided, I gathered some wood and built an altar with a little wooden cross in it. I started praying to Jesus and asking him to help me to get on a hockey team. Like most French families at the time, we were raised Catholic, and we went to church every Sunday. The church had given me a small red New Testament, and I had read the whole book. Every Easter, I would watch the Jesus movie and be so moved. My favorite Bible parable was Matthew

25:14–30. At nine years old, I understood that if God gave me five talents and if I used them, they would become ten talents. For that reason, it was very simple to me; I enjoyed hockey and sports, playing the violin, camping, and playing in the woods, skiing with my dad, and, yes, teasing my brothers and sisters. I also did fairly well in school even if it wasn't as much fun. In short, if I did five things the best I could, then I would be able to do ten things well; I did not know that talent was a form of money in biblical times. Very simple—I was a very happy child, with great parents.

But. Jesus, why doesn't Papa let me play hockey in the league?

As I became calm, I noticed how beautiful it was. The sun was shining through the canopy, and birds were chirping.

Oh no! I forgot to tell my parents where I was, I realized with dread, and I ran all the way home. When I got there, I abruptly stopped, opened the back door quietly, tiptoed in, and turned around to gently close the door.

"*Where have you been?*" my dad asked in an angry, fatherly voice that makes a kid tremble.

"I went for a walk!" I responded.

"You know to tell us where you go at all times!" he said.

"Well, I forgot! What's the big deal? You're the one who won't let me play hockey!"

I was staring at him, knowing full well that I was starting to irk him. *Jesus was quickly forgotten; now it was all about making it hard on my dad. Revenge was sweet!*

As things quickly escalated and I refused to discuss anything in a mature way, my dad had no choice but to ground me.

"*Go to your room!*" he angrily stated.

"*No!* Spank me! You always put me in my room, and Dan gets spanked, and that's over in two seconds! Spank me!"

My dad approached me and said, "Go to your room *now!*"

"*No.*"

My dad grabbed my arm and pulled me down the stairs and took me into my bedroom and said angrily "you will stay in your room for two days" and closed the door, not in a quiet way!

Later that day, as I sat angrily on my bed, I heard some laughter in our neighbor's, the Lemay's, yard. I glanced out my window and saw the Maisonneuves playing soccer. It looked like so much fun that I started to think that I could unlock my window, slide it open, and sneak out to play soccer for a little while and then sneak back in like nothing had ever happened. My bedroom was located in the basement, and the window was less than a foot above the ground.

As I proceeded with my plan and I was halfway out, I glanced up; there was my dad watching me from his bedroom window located just above mine! As you can guess—that didn't go so well at the time. But later in my adult life, that had become my dad's favorite story to share when I would visit him with my children and my husband.

I smiled remembering that event! I still believed that with my talent, I could do anything I wanted if I put in the hard work, but God was definitely out of the picture! Now it was me, myself, and I. Well, I always had playing hockey as a backup plan; however, right now, in the present, the best way to have success in soccer as a senior was to train with the best. And the best were UNC players and the UNC coach, Anson Dorrance, who also coached the women's national team.[1]

Nervously, I paced up and down my dorm room, stopped and sat down, picked up the phone, and dialed the UNC women's team number.

Maybe no one will pick up the phone, I thought.

"Hello! Anson Dorrance!"

"This is Fab Gareau! I play for NC State, and I would like to work for you in your summer camp. I heard that you have soccer training sessions also!" I blurted out without taking a breath.

He laughed! With mischief in his voice, he said, "*Gareau!* We would love to have you work with us, and yes, you can join our practices, and we also have pick-up games. It's a lot of fun!" He gave me all the information and the times to show up.

"Thank you so much!" I blurted. "I will be there and look forward to it!"

Working soccer camps at UNC was incredible! The summer after my sophomore year, I also worked camps for John Ellis, Jill

Ellis's father. Like Jill, he had helped coach the US women's soccer team. John Ellis was also a former Royal Marine Commando and had coached English club teams and now ran his own soccer academy and his own soccer camps in VA.[2] After training with Jill and then her father, I was about to work with the best coach and players in the world!

At UNC camp, first thing in the morning, Coach Anson Dorrance would run minipractices with the UNC players, me, and some other girls, some of whom were also on the national team. Here I was playing one-on-one against some of the best players in the world, if not the best two players in the world, Mia Hamm and Chris Lilly. One of my favorite memories was when Anson wanted to show coaches and players how to train female players to play more aggressively.

Anson announced, "Fab and Lil, you will both demonstrate! Fab, this is where you're only allowed to pull on the jerseys or shirts—you are not allowed to push while you possess the ball. You understand?"

"Got it."

Lil and I faced each other—stared at each other was more like it—with a soccer ball in between us as we waited for the whistle. When Anson blew the whistle, we both ejected forward like on springs and fought and fought for the ball. It was a constant battle, and we took turns pulling each other on the ground, barely touching the ball. It was vicious! I heard my shirt rip. We heard a whistle, and Anson yelled, "*Stop!*"

I looked down, and my shirt was completely ripped up. I was practically in my sports bra. You have to remember that back in the day, players never showed their bra. I was smiling—this one was a tie! She had just beaten me in the previous battle where two players stood shoulder to shoulder, waiting for the whistle. On the whistle, whichever player puts their arm up on top of the other player's arm will always win the race to the ball. That was my first time ever, and she had beaten me without trouble. *But this battle was a tie!* I thought.

Working UNC camps was so much fun—where I had learned more skills with Jill and her father. At UNC, I was also learning team tactics. I got to work with some of the best players and coaches in the country. Near the end of the week, I was exhausted: we had early sessions in the mornings and coached all day; at lunch break, we either scrimmaged each other or I worked on my shooting. Every night, someone bought some pizzas and, of course, beer was available if I was thirsty!

At the end of the week during our afternoon break, I grabbed a bag of balls and walked to the field by myself. The sun was beaming; it had to be high 90s in the early NC August summer. I felt hot, sweaty, and tired, but I wanted to work on my shooting before our NC State training camp started in a few weeks. I placed the balls in different areas of the field and started aiming in the corners, working on both my left and right foot. For the first time, I found myself asking, *Why does my right leg feel weak?* In the corner of my eye, I saw Anson Dorrance driving away. I kept going. *What's wrong with me? Why does my leg feel so weak? Why do I feel so tired?* I knelt down, then I slowly collected the balls and walked back. When I arrived at my room, I collapsed in my bed and rested. *Maybe—no more beer and pizza! Maybe—I will take a few days off, and my leg will get better. I have to make sure to eat healthier until the season starts!*

A few weeks later, I was on a different campus wearing red instead of Carolina blue and was surrounded by a rambunctious bunch of girls laughing, being glad to be back together again with my Wolfpack. It was the first day of training camp my senior year at the end of August 1991. In the early morning, the air was already full of humidity—it was going to be a normal, hot North Carolina summer, a warm day. We were divided into two groups on the track to be tested on how far we could run our twelve-minute run. UNC had to run a minimum of seven and a half laps, which was close to two miles in twelve minutes. That is fast for women! We only had to run seven laps. Over the years, I had developed a system! I hated long-distance running or any kind of running! I preferred for my fitness to play soccer or any sports for hours until I dropped. So I had bought a watch that I could program to beep at the end of each lap; this way, I would run exactly seven laps, no more, no less!

That session was the hardest twelve-minute run I had ever done! I felt so tired and weak, and every lap, I fell behind my beeps. With everything I had, I sprinted through the last part of the last lap and finished just in time. I was bent over, breathing hard, trying to catch my breath. My lungs felt like they were going to explode! *What is wrong with me? Why is my right leg so tight!*

After the UNC camp, I took it easy for two weeks. Something was wrong with my right hip/leg, and I felt tired! I decided not to worry because I was sure that I would become fit quickly with two practices a day in the following week, hoping to rebuild my strength! And everything was going to work out—this was my senior year! I had put in all the hard work and training for many years, and I felt confident that it was going to be a great year!

Wrong! It got worse and worse!

On October 3, 1991, halfway through the season, we were playing Methodist on the most beautiful field, the grass thick like a soft carpet.[3] I was not as excited to play this game because I always enjoyed playing against stronger opposition. *Maybe that was why I didn't have a pep in my step,* I reasoned. However, as the game progressed, my body felt worse and worse. My right leg was not working, and I felt so exhausted, like I had mono again. Eventually, Jill placed a perfect ball behind the defenders for me to run through using my quickness. I may not have been the fastest player, but I was usually the quickest one on the field. When we had been tested for the forty-yard dash on the Canadian National Team, I had the best time! But today was a different story—I could barely run, barely jog, and was so tired. I threw myself on the ground! I was physically and emotionally unable to push myself anymore—I was done! They blew the whistle, and I felt like a quitter as the trainer ran on the field.

"What's wrong? What happened? I didn't see anything!"

"I don't know! I feel so tired! It feels like I have mono again, and my right leg won't move anymore—it's so tight and heavy! I can't run anymore."

The trainer was a tall, big guy, and he helped me up, holding my arm, then I gently pushed his arm away and walked off the field with him. What torture—the game was on hold, and everyone was staring at me: the players, referees, coaches, and fans! I felt like the biggest loser, a quitter!

Who quits and walks off in the middle of a game? What's this shit? I'm the kind of player who gives 120%. What's wrong with me?

I collapsed on the bench as I was bombarded by questions from well-meaning coaches and players, who had become my friends, who shared everything in my life at the time. We battled together—we were like a pack of wolves, red wolves. But just then, like a wounded wolf, I just wanted to hide in my cave and be a lone wolf. I just told them that I agonized on why I couldn't run anymore and immediately transformed into a hermit.

Monday morning, the phone rang, and I knew it was my coach, and I told him that I would be right there. I walked to his office and collapsed in the chair, mentally and physically spent.

"Fab, what is wrong with you? Are you hurt?" He wanted to know.

"I don't know," I replied as I shrugged my shoulders. I truly had no idea, and I was baffled.

"This is your senior year, and you are having your worst season, and I have been very close to benching you. You are not running as fast or as much. You are not scoring either! Is it your new boyfriend?"

I exploded. "My boyfriend has nothing to do with this, and I would never let a guy stop me from playing sports. I would never have a boyfriend who doesn't support my sports!"

"Then tell me what's wrong and help me understand—no one knows what is going on." He was staring at me, waiting for me to respond.

"I don't know," the words came gushing out, and tears were rolling slowly down my cheeks. All the pent-up emotions came out! I explained how it had started in the summer and how I felt like I had mono again and how my right leg was not working. I couldn't really sprint anymore. Maybe it was a pinched nerve. *My leg was so weak and numb. My hip was so tight. I was so tired. I didn't know*! I usually never showed my emotions and tears like this, but I felt so hopeless and lost.

The next day, I started a regimen of tests and treatments. I had my first MRI to check my spine and my hip area, but everything appeared to be normal. I was given some strong anti-inflammatory meds and received a lot of treatments in the training room on a daily basis. I was also advised to get a shot of corticosteroids in my right side to remove the inflammation, but I refused with the advice of my mom who was a nurse! She had described to me the various side effects that could be harmful to me. If I had known at the time that it was my last chance to extend my athletic career, I would have said, "*Shoot me with as much corticosteroids as needed to enable me to play!*"

In addition to medicine and treatments, my new boyfriend, John Rudolph, was the best help! I had met him the previous spring semester as I was walking on campus with Suzie, one of my teammates. This bright-red sports car, a Pontiac Fiero, had pulled up beside us, and the window rolled down. This guy with the amazing blue eyes was looking at us and started talking to Suzie. I thought he sounded like that show *The Dukes of Hazzard* with his very strong Southern accent!

When we departed, I asked Suzie, "What's his name?"

"John! We have several classes together. He's in the same program as us."

Later in the week, I rushed to my new class, late as usual. I was not a morning person, and I would always get up at the last minute and jog to class. Once there, I hurried to the only available desk in the classroom, and to my surprise, I noticed that he was sitting behind me. As I sat down, I smiled shyly at him and said "hi" and turned around to face the teacher. As the teacher rambled on and on, I slid down my seat and rested my head back and closed my eyes. All of sudden, I became very uncomfortable as I realized that my hair was all over his desk!

Following that event, I would see him everywhere! Suzie and I ended up playing football with him and his friends, and then we casually went to get a bite of fast food. That weekend, we were invited to a party where most of my teammates were present. And there he was again! We ended up talking to each other all night, like it was just the two of us there! Later, when we were dating, he admitted to me that he had been playing with my hair on that first day in class! His response to my protest was "You should not have put your curly hair all over my desk!"

Who would have known at the time that he was going to become my husband and the father of my two children: Melissa and Tristan. At the time, he was so good to me as I was struggling with my soccer! Almost every day, he would massage my stiff leg and especially on game days. That, along with the other treatments, led to better games. Unfortunately, my senior year was almost over!

On Sunday, November 10, 1991, we were playing the University of Central Florida in the NCAA first round,[3] just like my freshman year. I felt good—just like my freshman year! I was full of energy, and my leg was working, and I scored two goals in that game.[4] I was feeling it! I was also feisty like my old self. Their defender kept kicking me on the back of my calves, and I had had enough!

As she was kicking me one more time, I turned around and punched her in the face and kept running like nothing had happened so the referee would not notice! From the corner of my eye, I realized that she was chasing me like a raging bull and cursing at me and calling me *not so nice names*! I stopped, and thinking that I would be playing UNC the next week, I threw myself on the ground and covered my face and head as she was pounding me.[4] The thought of not getting ejected from the game occurred in a fraction of a second. *I cannot fight back so I don't get thrown out for the last game against UNC in the quarter finals*!

Jody, our tall defender, sprinted down the field and pulled her off me. That's my teammate! That defender ended up getting a red card later in the game and getting ejected.[4] She got kicked out, and I got to play against UNC the following week! I was so pumped and ready to play UNC one last time! I was so excited!

One week later, I was sitting in the bus with my Wolfpack team on my way to Chapel Hill. It was a quiet bunch; everyone was so focused on the task at hand. Most girls were listening to motivating music on their Walkmans! Just like all the games through my collegiate career, we walked to our bench when we arrived and went through our warm-up while the stadium filled up with a crowd dressed in Carolina blue.

Unlike the previous game, unlike the last five years, it was a disaster! We got hammered, 4–1![5] My body was not working again—

once so quick, now so slow…once so full of energy, now so tired…once so feisty, now so beaten down…born a super athlete, now reduced to nothing.

I once, as an eight-year-old, told my mom that I would be in the Olympics! I had dreamed of being in the World Cup, the Olympics, or playing professionally or all three—I believed that deep in my soul!

If that is all taken away from me, who am I? Once, I was living my dream. Now I am a loser, now I am depressed!

Part 2

Lost

CHAPTER 5

Diagnosis

Nine and a half years later, on Monday, April 23, 2001, I was sitting at my computer, working on engineering drawings for my father-in-law, who was a civil engineer. A few years earlier, I had bought a book with several tutorials to self-learn computer drafting. I did this so I could stay home to raise my daughter, Melissa. I wanted to be home to cherish every milestone in her young life from the baby stage until she started school! And when my son, Tristan, was born two and half years later, I did the same for him. They were both so special to me! It was my way of attempting to move on with life, happily married and content. I had two great, healthy children and a loving husband!

As I sat and pondered about my family, my pain reached a new level! It was agonizing! I hunched over with my head resting in my hands. I couldn't take it anymore! The pain was excruciating. My headache was like nothing I had ever experienced before, and this had been going on for two weeks, but now vision in my right eye was also blurred. I couldn't see my computer screen—it was fuzzy! My husband walked into the room.

"What's wrong?"

"What's wrong? You're not helping me enough! I have to take care of the kids, clean the house, and then work on the computer, and I'm exhausted!" I was unfairly screaming at him, taking it out on him, and I burst out crying.

John rushed over, put his arms around me, and held me tightly.

"What's wrong?" he asked with concern in his voice.

I straightened my head and looked at him with tears rolling down my face.

"I'm scared! I've had a headache for two weeks, and it keeps getting worse, and now I can't see with my right eye. It's blurry!"

John called his mom to make sure that my in-laws could take care of the kids the following day and drive them to school and pre-school while I made an appointment with an ophthalmologist for the following day.

On the next day, when I was sitting in a medical room and the doctor had just finished examining my right eye, she looked at me and said, "You have optic neuritis. That means that your optic nerve is very swollen and inflamed. You either have cancer or MS, short for multiple sclerosis!"

I was speechless.

"I would like you to go see a neurologist and also get an MRI. My brother, Dr. Price, is a neurologist in Greenville, North Carolina, and I can get you an appointment today."

Again, I was speechless as we were driving to Greenville for my next appointment, and John didn't say a word either! It was a very quiet ride involving two very scared individuals.

After two days of various doctors and tests, including a brain MRI and a lumbar puncture, Dr. Price told both of us that I had lesions in my brain and that I probably had MS. At that time, doctors didn't diagnose MS until a person had two exacerbations known as flare-ups. According to the National MS Society, an exacerbation of MS (also known as a relapse, attack, or flare-up) is the occurrence of new symptoms or the worsening of old symptoms. It can be very mild or severe enough to interfere with a person's ability to function.

John asked, "What exactly is MS?"

Dr. Price described how MS stands for multiple sclerosis and how my own immune system was attacking my brain and my nervous system. He also listed the various symptoms. "They are fatigue, vision problems, numbness and tingling, muscle spasms, stiffness and weakness, pain, just to name a few symptoms. Some of which you already have! Additionally, the majority of MS patients are in a wheelchair within twenty years!"

"The good news is it's not cancer!" he also said.

The last two days were so exhausting to me, and the headaches were so excruciating that I barely reacted. I just wanted to go home to rest. I was so overwhelmed with fatigue and pain that it never occurred to me that John also had to be struggling with this.

That same evening, I was lying down on the floor in the den, quietly watching TV because I couldn't sleep. I was still in pain from the lumbar puncture and headache, even after all the painkillers they had administered to me. To my surprise, as I was switching channels, a TV host came on the air and said, "My name is Montel Williams, and I have multiple sclerosis![1] Let me tell you my story and how I was diagnosed two years ago!"

Oh crap! What a coincidence!

Then he proceeded to tell his story about being in the Marines, having problems with his legs, numbness and pain, and enduring all the tests he had been given, but because he was so fit and physically strong, he was always told it was probably just a pinched nerve.

"It will go away with rest and anti-inflammatories!" they had told him.

Finally, he was diagnosed with MS when he experienced vision problems with optic neuritis.

That's me! That is so me!

Slowly, my head was showered with flashbacks! For the last nine and a half years, my life had been like a yo-yo, up and down. The first thing I did after my collegiate career was to retire from the national team because I could no longer play at that highest level.

During that time, I would train and get fit and then try to play, only to crash again and again! For instance, a semipro soccer team for women was started in the summer of 1994 to play in a new league. We were called the Greensboro Dynamo. It was a team packed with talent and included four US national team players, Mia Ham, Carla Werden-Overbeck, Wendy Gebauer, and Tisha Venturini. In addition, the rest of the team was fielded with retired players from Duke, NC State, and UNC. It was stacked![2] And my yo-yo career kept on!

For example, one weekend, I scored two goals on Saturday, and the next day, on Sunday, I couldn't run because my right hip and leg would be so tight, numb, and weak. To this day, I remember Anson Dorrance asking me, "Why didn't you play the same way on Sunday?" Also, in one of our practices, Carla Overbeck, the best sweeper in the world at the time, asked me if she could be paired up against me in our fitness sprints because I was known to be the quickest player. We were working on our quickness and explosion with shorts sprints. When we raced, we were even or she beat me.

After practice, I asked Dino, our coach and also the UNC assistant coach, "How come I lost my quickness? Also, my right leg and my hip are so weak. I can't figure out what is going on!"

He responded, "It's because you haven't played in a long time—you will build it back up."

"*No! Something is wrong!*" I wanted to scream.

In another fitness session, we were doing intervals on the whole field, and if one player did not finish in the allotted time, the whole group had to rerun all the intervals. Guess who couldn't finish on time? Me! Guess who was watching? Anson! *What an embarrassment!*

After our summer season was over, we entered our team in the nationals, and we represented North Carolina. We flew to Texas for the regionals. I was playing upfront with Mia Hamm, known as the best player in the world. Again, my body failed me, and I was taken out of the first game after fifteen minutes. Later in the game, he put me back in, and a perfect ball was crossed in the box, and I made my diagonal run at full speed and jumped to head the ball in. However, I could no longer jump off the ground and ended up scoring with the top of my head in a very weird way.

When I was subbed off, Dino was laughing and asked me, "Did you always head the ball with the top of your head?"

"No, I headed it with my forehead!" I lied, and I wanted to hide and disappear.

Of all the ups and downs of that nine-and-a-half-year period, the worst one occurred when I received a phone call in 1995 from a Japanese soccer coach. He told me that Anson Dorrance had given him my name because he was trying to find a player to play for them. I knew many collegiate players including Charmaine and Jill, who were playing there. The Japanese clubs would provide the girls with a car and a place to stay in addition to their salary. For a second, my heart was beating fast with excitement, but just as quickly, reality hit me.

With doubt in my voice, I answered him, "I'm sorry! I cannot play soccer right now because I am pregnant, but I can play for you after the baby is born!"

We hung up, and I never heard from him again.

It was not for a lack of trying that I didn't go play in Japan. After Melissa was born, I would push her in the stroller to Fairfield Park in Kinston, North Carolina, where we lived at the time. I would make sure that she was shaded enough in the bright North Carolina sun while I worked on some dribbling, and at the same time, I would be talking to her. Once she fell asleep, I would work on my fitness and sprints. Same old, same old—the first day, I would feel normal, and as I continued the following days, it would get worse and worse.

Again, in 1997, I saw a neurologist for my weakness and numbness in my right leg. The MRI of my spine showed nothing wrong, and I was prescribed diclofenac and rest to reduce the inflammation.

On and on and on like a yo-yo, now I remembered as I was listening to Montel Williams and lying on the floor, all drugged up with painkillers. Montel Williams had just finished describing the same thing that had happened to him.

I have MS. I'm not crazy!

"John!" I yelled, "John, come here!"

"Is something wrong?" he asked, all worried. "Are you okay?"

"Yes, I'm fine! I have MS. Look, Montel Williams has MS, and he wasn't diagnosed either because he was so strong and fit like me!"

"No, Dr. Price said maybe you don't have it. It's not definite yet."

My husband, John, didn't want to believe that the active woman whom he had fallen in love with and who used to play soccer with him, hike, camp, and surf, to name a few activities, would end up in a wheelchair! I let it go, but I knew I had MS. I had felt it the last nine and half years, and I also knew that nothing would have stopped me from doing my sports. As selfish as it might have been, I was even ready to fly to Japan with my daughter! Only something as serious as MS could stop me.

CHAPTER 6

Help Me, Help Me

As much as I was thankful to finally know what it was, it didn't get any easier—*it got harder, much harder.* Looking back at my medical records, I visited the doctor's fifteen times in that first year to try different medicines, throwing up on the first two meds with my liver enzyme dangerously spiking up. That didn't even include the times I had to receive the steroid medicine intravenously and dealing with the side effects, anger, facial hair, and not sleeping. Then I had another flare-up! For the second time, my symptoms increased instantly and exponentially! Full-blown MS invaded my close-to-normal life! Furthermore, it was devastating personally to observe the disruption in the lives of the people whom I loved most!

My eyes were slowly improving, but the computer screen was not completely clear. All of a sudden, my right arm was weak, and I couldn't use the mouse anymore. *No problem, I will use my left hand to control the mouse,* which I learned to do. Then, in addition to my right leg being weak and numb, my other leg became weak.

My three-year-old son, Tristan, ran up to me with a book.

"Maman, Maman," he said and jumped in my arms!

Yes, at the time, I still talked to my kids in French! He was a very active little boy. I caught him in my arms, and we both fell. My legs and my arms were too weak to hold him. Acting like it was just a game and we were meant to fall, I grabbed the book to read to him. It was blurry! I could not read him the story!

When Tristan's attention quickly turned to another toy, I lay there holding all my emotions in. I had just realized that I had just lost the last, important thing to me: taking care of my children, Melissa and Tristan. I had already lost my sports, now I couldn't work, and John hired Mike to do the computer drafting! I couldn't be a wife! Now I couldn't take care of my children! Melissa was being taken care of by my in-laws, and John was taking care of Tristan. *I had completely hit rock bottom.* Suicidal thoughts crossed my mind, and depression hit me like a strong hurricane. I kept everything to myself until that night.

When we finally went to bed, I kept tossing and turning, feeling so hopeless and depressed. I slowly made it to the couch and laid there. I started crying softly to not wake anyone. Then it slowly got louder and louder and louder. Loud cries turned to sobs, and I screamed to the top of my lungs, "*God, help*! *God, help*! *God, help*!

The sobbing got louder. Then, for some reason, without thinking, maybe because I was raised Catholic, I said, "Jesus, if you are real, help me!"

To this day, I have never again prayed two words so desperately: "*God, help.*"

Soon after, I was alone with John, trying to share my feelings of hopelessness, but I had never been very good at expressing myself, and I had never felt so weak and useless. To my surprise, as I was trying to express my desperation, John erupted like a volcano and started venting and yelling and throwing his surveying equipment everywhere! That equipment is super expensive, thousands of dollars. John was the most incredible husband to me. He had passed his surveying license and started his own company with no cash flow, which was so impressive to me. The business was just starting to be profitable! *That was the moment I realized that he too had just hit rock bottom.*

It just occurred to me that everything he had just built in two years, a successful business, he had just lost in one month. He was not working but taking care of Tristan. We had been living on credit cards—it didn't even occur to us to ask his parents to help us financially! His parents were already taking care of Melissa. We were two strong-minded individuals *until we both hit rock-bottom, until that one moment.* We lay on the floor, holding each other, with tears in our eyes, both feeling hopeless!

Two things here are important. *First,* an autoimmune or serious illness will knock you out so hard that you can hardly breathe; it will rob you of your dreams. It will not only hurt you but it will also change the lives of all your loved ones around you. Can you imagine a parent watching his or her child go through something like that? My mom flew from Canada in that time to help us, and I still remember the sadness and pain in her eyes as she was watching me. Can you envision the spouse who fell in love with his loved one who used to be so active and full of life but no longer? Can you also picture the child who, all of a sudden, is being taken care of by the grandparents?

"Where is Mommy?" they would ask.

"Mommy is sick," they were told.

When I looked back at my medical chart, the doctor had written: "The patient might need a psychiatrist to deal with her depression, and her daughter is also struggling with her illness."

Second, in the midst of all that suffering and that pain, in the lowest point of your life when you are ready to give up, to not live, when you feel like you are just a burden for your loved ones and that they would be better off without you, God hears your most desperate cry in the middle of the night: "*God, help!*"

When the strong-willed person who believes that he or she can accomplish anything and everything he or she wants, when that person is completely beat down and, in desperation, cries out: "*God, help!*"

God can now help that person! That person no longer relies on himself or herself. That person needs help. And God who has been right there beside you, waiting to help you, *can now take over.*

Do you believe in miracles?

CHAPTER 7

God Heard Me

AT ABOUT THAT TIME, I BEGAN TO slowly get better. My vision also came back, and I started a search for God!

"Desperate times call for desperate measures," they say.

I was taking my kids to the library to get them books, and they also loved Story Time, when the librarian would read a story to the little kids! I started reading about Islam and its history, and very quickly, I decided Islam wasn't for me.

Next, I started researching Buddhism. One time, I was trying to meditate, humming, "Hmmm! Hmmm!" Melissa came running in the room and busted out laughing.

"What are you doing?"

"I'm trying to do meditation like Buddhist monks," I answered her.

"Can I try? Let me try!"

We both sat on the floor, Indian style, with our eyes closed, in her bedroom and started, "Hmmm! Hmmm!" And we both opened our eyes, looked at each other, and cracked up laughing, and we had the best time just laughing nonstop.

According to Buddhism, I could be incarnated into anything in my second life. For instance, I could become an ant, and when I entered someone's home, they could squish me! On the other side of it, Buddhist monks had a hard time killing ants during an infestation in their monastery because they could be incarnated people! Nonsense! Buddhism wasn't for me!

At that time, we lived in Kinston, North Carolina, and every day, I would take walks with my kids in the stroller. Of course, Melissa would always jump out and strongly declare that I was walking, and I smiled!

I wonder where she gets that grit!

Slowly, over time, four women—Gayla, Diane, Beth, and Julie—would talk to me as I walked by, and then, eventually, they invited me in their playgroup, where each one took turns to take care of the kids while the other women took half a day off. It was great! Here and there, they would invite me to their church or a Christian concert. Or they would invite John and Melissa and Tristan and I for supper. After being invited for a Christian outing, I would always go home and laugh with John.

"They are trying to convert me," I'd say, and we would both laugh.

Later, Ashely joined the group, and we developed a friendship. *Let me stop you right here, Christians!* Christians, it is not your preaching and quoting the Bible to unbelievers that will make a difference in their lives, especially when they are hurting. I was hurting. I still wanted to be a professional athlete. These women became my friends and shared their lives and their children with me. I was not a Christian, but I respected them. I told my husband they didn't just talk the talk; they walked the walk!

Ashely took over and invited me to her home for many lunches and kept my children many times to help me out. When she was pregnant with her youngest son, Parker, she was bedridden for most of the pregnancy. She invited the younger school children from our school to do the Easter egg hunt in her backyard! That was so impressive to me—what an amazing woman! How do you open your home for these children when you are bedridden and you don't even know if your child will be normal? That was when I, as an unbeliever, started wondering, *Where does that strength come from? How can she be so unselfish? How is that possible? How are they so loving?*

It was one of those times when I was having lunch in Ashely's home that she saw my library books, including books on Buddhism.

We started talking about religion, and she told me about her faith in Jesus Christ.

I told her, "Ashely, I know all about Christianity, about Jesus Christ! I was raised Catholic! I went to church every Sunday!"

"But do you know him intimately?"

"I did when I was young, but now I don't know if Jesus is real. I need proof. I need to know that he is truly God and truly resurrected."

And she responded, "I will be right back."

She hurried upstairs, hurried back down, and gave me a book called *More Than a Carpenter* by Josh McDowell. It's a small book explaining with reliable facts, history, and Bible verses why Jesus is truly God and that he was truly resurrected. I went home to read that book. Then I read the simple prayer in the back of the book! I read the prayer and asked Jesus to forgive me, and I gave my life to Jesus. In that instant, a warmth and tingling feeling took over my body as I was lying in bed before going to sleep.

That was the beginning of my young Christian life, which I chronicled in a journal. That warmth and tingling feeling just was not enough for me! As a consequence, I read Josh McDowell's bigger book, *Evidence That Demands a Verdict*. This detailed book provides a strong defense of Christianity's truths and rebuttals to skeptics, with strong evidence for Jesus, the Bible, the Old Testament, and the Truth.

When I informed John about what happened to me, he also read the book *More Than a Carpenter*. Another perspective captured him. For him, a man who loves history, he said, "That is so true. In war, when the men go through torture, there's always one man that will break! But none of the apostles broke down or changed their stance on the resurrection!"

That night, he prayed that same prayer in the back of the book. In the morning, he told me all about it!

"Did you have a small tingling?" I asked.

"No, I had nightmares all night long, and it was very scary!"

Yet John and I were continuing on our adventure through our life together.

Shortly after, as a new Christian and not knowing much except for a little tingling, I was doubting again because of my health. I felt miserable! I asked God, "God, give me a sign that believing in you is the right thing to do!"

I was watching *The 700 Club*, a Christian show that always had a five-minute segment where the hosts prayed healing on different people and conditions, and that was my hope and the only reason I watched it. The segment came on, and the host said, "Someone out there, you have turned to Jesus, but you're starting to doubt again, but God wants you to hang in there!" Yes, you might say that this is very generic, but I just started crying! It spoke to me!

A couple of days later, I was feeling so sick, and I was so exhausted. I had lost some of our keys and dragged myself everywhere, searching for the keys. As I was searching and then getting ready to go to the car dealership to get some car keys made, I prayed, "God, you know I can't handle this right now. Please just help me find our keys."

As I was searching and praying, my inner voice, or at least I thought it was my inner voice, kept saying over and over, "Go do a load of laundry." That did not make sense to me because I certainly didn't have the energy to do laundry.

I dragged myself to our other car, drove to the car dealership, and got some keys made! Sure enough, on the weekend, John said, "Guess what I found when I was doing laundry—the keys on the washing machine!"

I realized, *I should have listened to God!*

I was a baby Christian—how would I have known—I thought it was my inner voice! It never crossed my mind that it could be God.

In April 2002, Ashely called me on the phone.

"Hey, Fab, you want to go to a conference in Raleigh, North Carolina, this weekend? It's Anne Graham Lotz. She's the sister of Billy Graham.[1] I have an extra ticket, and I already have hotel reservations."

"Let me think about it and see if I can, and I will call you back later."

I didn't really want to go. I was still feeling miserable, but I told myself if John would tell me to go, I would go. I was so sure he would tell me "that's stupid" or not care, but John surprised me.

"I think that's a great idea! It would be really good for you to get out!"

So I called her back and agreed to meet her there in our hotel room.

The day of the event, I was a little excited! John had agreed to keep the kids for two days, and I was going somewhere out of the house for two days.

John was right, I thought. *This will be nice to get away and be with friends!*

As I was thinking about all this, I peeked in the mirror and noticed how tired I looked, and I thought, *Oh no! I can't go like this*—my face was full of facial hair, black hair, like I had never seen before. And I remembered that it was one of the side effects of the prescription of prednisone I had just finished.

I headed to the store, bought some hair removal cream, came back home, and went to work. To my dismay, when I was through, my face was all red, very red. I had a chemical reaction to it.

"*John*! Look at my face," I cried, and I explained what had happened.

"Don't worry! It will go away by the time you get there!" he assured me.

I listened to his advice, finished packing, and headed to Raleigh, North Carolina, a one-and-a-half-hour drive from Kinston, where we lived at the time.

When I got there, I didn't waste time. I arrived early before the rest of the group, checked in, and, right away, took my bathing suit out of my soccer bag. I had just read that swimming was really good for people with MS, and it felt like I hadn't exercised in so long! This was exciting! I walked slowly to the pool, jumped in with a smile, and just started swimming.

Oh, that feels great!

I was full of adrenaline, swimming on and on, getting all my rage out of my system; all my new frustrations of my new life went out the door. And I pushed some more! It felt great!

Completely exhausted, I reached the end of the pool, stopped, and leaned my back on the side of the pool! I felt great and tired!

When was the last time I worked out this hard? I wondered as I grinned.

Then I noticed that my eyes were killing me because I had swum without goggles. I headed back to the room so I would have time to shower and hopefully get the chlorine out of my eyes.

When I finally came out of the shower and finished dressing up, I looked in the mirror, and I was horrified! I looked horrible! I looked sick, like a very sick woman! My face was still red from the reaction to the hair removal, my eyes were bloodshot and burning from the chlorine, and I looked like I felt super tired.

What am I doing here? I wondered.

As I was thinking of leaving, I heard the door opening, and Ashely came in.

"Hi, I'm so glad you came. This is going to be fun!"

She was so bubbly, and I sure wasn't. And I started explaining why my face and eyes were all messed up.

"Fab, everything will work out! Don't worry! We will find someone with eye drops to relieve the soreness of your eyes."

Ashely was always the one to encourage you, and I sure needed that at the time!

After welcoming all the women in the group and eating some supper, we headed to the hockey arena, now known as PNC Stadium. Once seated, I looked around me, and I was amazed that it was full, mostly all women.

Anne Graham Lotz spoke about God, about Jesus, and then some singers took over. It was amazing! I had goose bumps; the place was full of the Holy Spirit. The singers started playing more softly, and Anne spoke in the microphone to invite any one to come to the altar and invite Jesus in your heart and in your life. I had already done that one night in my bed, but I felt led to do it again publicly this time! That in itself was incredible! For me to do that publicly was very unlike me! As much as I thought that this was amazing, I had no idea that *God was going to blow me away the next day*!

The next day, I was seated with Ashely's friend in the arena, away from the rest of the group. The guest speaker came on, and the theme of her session was on how to pray. She said, "Close your eyes and picture Jesus has his hands on each side of your face and says he loves you." I never heard anything she said after that! I then experienced the most incredible phenomenon I have ever experienced in my whole life! I felt Jesus's hands on my face. I felt his presence and his power. I didn't really see him, but I felt his love and power. It was all around me and in me, and there was kind of a light, white light, that I had never seen or experienced before! I was alone with Jesus! I kept trying to ask him, "Why did you give me such talent and then take it away?"

But he would never let me finish, and he would interrupt me by saying gently, "I love you!"

And again, I would say, "Why did you give me such talent and then take it away?"

"I love you," he would interrupt me gently again!

And on and on, we went on back and forth.

At the same time, my pain, my innermost pain, from the last ten years of being unable to live my dreams because of my MS was flowing out of me and being replaced with his love. So much love was pouring in; so much pain was leaving! I'm not sure how long it lasted—it could have been two minutes or two hours!

Then I realized that I was crying like a baby, and I wasn't alone. I opened my eyes, and the place was full of women singing. I tried to stop crying, but that feeling was still occurring while my eyes were open! So I just closed my eyes and surrendered back to Jesus's love! But Jesus had left! I knew he was still with me, but I could no longer feel his hands and see his light physically, but I knew, without a shadow of doubt, that he was real.

To this day, that innermost, deep pain has never come back. I was healed that day from that suffering pain, unfulfilled dreams, and physical and emotional pain that was so deep. The deep pain had just flowed out, and Jesus's love flowed in!

On the drive home from Raleigh, I was so emotionally and physically exhausted! My face had been red from the reaction of the hair remover chemicals, and my eyes were still burning and red. The drive was difficult; my legs were burning and in pain, symptoms of MS. On the contrary, I had been healed of all my deepest emotional pain and seen the white light, the love of Jesus all around me, all in me! I could not wait to be home and tell John and share the best experience of my life!

I came in all excited and exclaimed in an excited voice, "Hey, John!"

"How was your weekend?" he said as he hugged me.

With the biggest smile on my face, I said in a voice full of life and excitement, "It was so amazing!" And I recounted all that had happened to me and my encounter with Jesus Christ.

"That's nice," he said as he moved on to doing what he was doing.

In an instant, I felt hurt! I had been on a high, full of Jesus. Now I was so deflated. I had been on the mountain; now I was in the valley! I had just assumed that my husband would share the same level of excitement and belief in Jesus. But he had not been there, instead keeping two young kids by himself! Understandably, he was tired!

Back to reality, I started living like a new Christian, full of hope! It was, at times, a lonely path but full of growth. I had slowly started reading my Bible, and I started going to church with my in-laws, and my children started attending Sunday school. For me, that was lonely at times because John still was not going to church! I wanted to share my hope and new belief in Christ with him so badly! So I followed 1 Peter 3:1–2, which, today, can be very controversial. It says: "Wives, in the same way submit yourselves to your own husbands so that, if any of them do not believe the word, they may be won over without words by the behavior of their wives, when they see the purity and reverence of their lives."

I realized in biblical times, married couples were different. To me, I was still going to respect and love my husband with all my heart and mind, no other man! I was not going to nag him anymore about going to church, and I was going to live my life in Jesus in a quiet manner and as an example. No more nagging!

One day, he said, "I want what you have!"

Eventually, he started going to church, got baptized, and was confirmed, along with both my children!

CHAPTER 8

Life or Death, You Choose

In February 2006, approximately four years later, I hit another low with my disease. The last four years had been an adjustment to accept MS, but life had become almost normal. It was normal family life with two young children.

In addition to work and school, we enjoyed the outdoors like camping, canoeing, hiking, and all things that I could still do. I also kept the kids entertained by going to the playground, library, movies. I could be very creative at times.

For example, I had found a purple-and-yellow house that I pretended was the Easter Bunny's house. We would park in the front of that house, but the Easter Bunny never came out! I love young children, and I could always come up with different activities.

My normal family life was abruptly interrupted when I became ill with the flu. I had grown accustomed to my leg numbness, cramps, and pain, but with this flu, it was turned up more than a notch. It spiraled up to almost unbearable! And every time that I had been sick, including colds, my joints would keep hurting for a month, often longer. I started really thinking as I was lying in bed. *If joint pain is unbearable at thirty-eight years old, how is it going to be at fifty? At seventy? Older than that?* The joint pain was unbearable now, but all of sudden, I was thinking about pain like this or worse for five years, ten years, and thirty years, and I could not deal with that! I was unable to cope with that! I became suicidal!

For the second time in my life, I did not want to live! Dealing with an autoimmune disease can be difficult when you live life one day at a time. However, when you start imagining how it would be for thirty or forty years, it'd become unbearable. If pain, physical or emotional, was unbearable now, how could I live with such pain for thirty or forty years? Impossible!

Looking back, it was very simple to tell someone "you need to live one day at a time" or "it will come to pass—it won't always be like this!" But if you were in the midst of such pain, you could not see straight. You could not think normally because all you felt was pain.

For me, it was physical pain above what I could tolerate! But for you, it might be emotional, but it would be beyond your threshold! It could be drugs that you could not stop or a dangerous or hopeless situation where you saw no way out! At that point, *please seek help*! Reach out to anyone: a coworker, a friend, a family member, your preacher, God, or anyone listening to you. Likewise, if you observe a person depressed or struggling with suicidal thoughts, please help them! You could save a life!

I was beaten down! Again! This time, however, I had God and the Bible and prayer, but suicidal thoughts still invaded my head as I started looking in the Bible for anything relating to suicides. I had to look it up because fears invaded my mind: *What happens if I kill myself? Could I go to hell? What if hell is worse than MS but for eternity, never ending!*

Nothing! I couldn't find a thing. I started researching death, but nothing that I found was talking about suicides! Finally, I looked up life, and as I started reading Deuteronomy 30:11–20, it was as if God was talking to me. In a nutshell, it said: "Now what I am commanding you today is not too difficult for you or beyond your reach…I have set before you life and death, blessings and curses. Now choose life…For the Lord is your life…"

A couple days later, I was helping Tristan clean his room because he had been sick also. He could tell that I was not feeling great myself, and he said, "Maman! You don't have to help if you feel bad."

I responded forcefully, "I don't do anything that I don't choose to do!"

"No, Maman! Sometimes, God asks something of us that is very difficult, but we have to do it because he asks us!"

I couldn't believe that he was just eight years old!

"Tristan, I think that God just used you to talk to me!"

And I explained to him what I had just read in the Bible.

He was so excited that he ran to Melissa's room and spoke excitedly, "Melissa! Melissa! I didn't know it, but God used me to talk to Maman! And I didn't know it!"

I walked to her room, and both of us explained to Melissa what had happened. Maybe that was what Jesus meant when he said for us to have faith like little children (Matthew 19:14). We were so excited!

Later that week, I received the CBN brochure, the Christian brochure that I read every month. I still wasn't feeling great, and for the first time, I threw it out! I was too busy, and I was barely surviving my day. However, I strongly felt like I should read it. I thought *I will just read the Pat Robertson part* as I picked it out of the garbage can. I slowly opened it up, and there it was: "I'm giving you a choice between life and prosperity, death and disaster…between life and death…" (Deuteronomy 30:15–16 NLT).

I absolutely knew that God was telling me to live. *God had just told me three times in one week to choose life*! To this day, I have not considered suicide again. God is my life! I was healed again from suicidal thoughts!

Part 3

Healing

CHAPTER 9

Healing with My Mom

In 2010, I had basically learned how to live with my MS. John and I were coaching Melissa's travel soccer team, and I could still scrimmage with the girls at the end of practice. To my standards of comparing to my past game, I was horrible, but thinking about it now, I should have been more thankful to have MS and still be able to run and kick a soccer ball.

Eventually, I ended up coaching at a local private school in Kinston, North Carolina called Arendell Parrott Academy also! I wasn't as crazy about coaching as playing, but the relationships that I had developed with the girls I will treasure for the rest of my life!

Four years after a normal family life, the Lord spoke to me again, this time for someone else.

In October of that year, John looked at me and asked, "Are you nervous about your mom coming? You are sure praying a lot."

I explained to him that I had been reading the French Bible and learning scriptures so I could talk to her about Jesus in French, but I kept feeling frustrated. Then the words from John 10:14 and John 10:16 jumped at me: "I am the Good Shepherd…I have other sheep that are not of this sheep pen. I must bring them also. They too will listen to my voice, and there shall be one flock and one shepherd."

I explained to John that I felt that God had given me that Word for my mom, and I kept praying it over her!

While my mom was visiting, after one of our talks, my mom exploded against Christianity and my beliefs and told me that evil did not exist. After calmly explaining my beliefs, I was baffled. I was so sure that God had given me that scripture for my mom! I told John what had happened, and he suggested that I lend her the book *More Than a Carpenter.*

The next morning, she agreed to read the book, and for lunch, I took her to the Village Green Steakhouse, a popular steakhouse located on Highway 70, Goldsboro, a five-minute drive from my house. We were having a good time, and my rare steak was succulent.

Out of the blue, she blurted out, "You want me to be honest? You want to know who I pray to?"

Without waiting for my answer, she continued, "God is my Good Shepherd, and I am his sheep."

Again, four years later, I was amazed that, indeed, I had heard from God. This was an amazing moment for me. When we arrived home, I showed her my French Bible and where I had underlined John 10:14 and 10:16 and written her name by it with the date 10/22/10. She also read *More Than a Carpenter* and said that it made sense to her.

Today, in the year 2023, I don't think that she is living for Christ, but God let me know that one day, she will!

CHAPTER 10

Gradual Decline, Gradual Healing

From that moment on, my physical ability slowly declined, sometimes so gradually that I didn't realize it until it was too late. I loved to run after my kids, but I soon realized that I had slowed down a lot when I could no longer catch Tristan! We would play tag on the playground, and I could no longer catch him.

One time, I was playing tag with both Melissa and Tristan in our yard. Melissa is a long-distance runner, and both Tristan and I are sprinters and faster.

When Melissa was it and couldn't catch us, she just ran behind us and said, "Don't worry, I will just keep running, and both of you will get tired, and I will eventually catch one of you."

That was the funniest thing. Tristan and I kept racing around the house with Melissa right behind us, and round and round we went. As we were getting tired, it was either Tristan or I who would slow down and would get caught. That time, it was Tristan! We were laughing so hard!

In middle school, when Melissa played travel soccer, I would scrimmage at the end of most practices with the girls and maintain my running ability. Then Melissa decided to stop playing travel and started playing for her school, Arendell Parrott Academy (APA).

Soon after APA asked me to coach the JV team, I realized I could no longer run for long periods of time because I had stopped running after I stopped coaching the travel team. Eventually, when my right leg was getting weaker, I started using my left leg to demonstrate different soccer skills. Then, one day, I realized I could no longer kick with my right leg. Near the end of my coaching career, I asked the best players to demonstrate when I could no longer do it.

The year 2016 was my last year coaching, and it was the hardest. By then, I was coaching both the JV girls and boys. I would work during the day and coach practice from three to five and on game days; sometimes, we wouldn't come home until 11:00 p.m. That year was a blur—I was always exhausted. Once practices were over, sometimes, I would sit in my vehicle for fifteen to thirty minutes to rest before I was able to drive home. After that season, I called Shivar, who was in charge of the soccer program, and told him I could no longer physically do it. That was one of the hardest, most emotional decisions I ever had to make. MS had finally, completely robbed me of soccer.

I have many memories of "dying to sports" that I loved, meaning on a particular day, I would notice that I could no longer perform a certain sport or physical activity. One instance happened in February 2014 when I flew home in the winter because my dad had been sick.

One day, we decided to play hockey on the neighborhood skating rink near Julie's, my sister's house. Her husband was in charge of maintaining the ice, and while he was clearing the snow off the ice, we all started getting ready and putting our skates on. Melanie, my younger sister, lent me her skates, and I was so excited to play with my siblings and some of my nieces and nephew and also my dad. Hockey is my favorite sport!

Once I finished putting on skates, I walked to the pile of hockey sticks and grabbed one. I walked to the ice, full of joy. I started skating and fell. I got up, and we started scrimmaging, and I fell and fell and fell, nonstop. My mom, my dad, and Melanie were begging me to stop, but I kept going. I just felt like crying. I knew this was my last time. I was dying to hockey. That is an expression that I made up to attempt to let it go and accept it.

On a different Canada winter trip in December 2017, we went downhill skiing and snowboarding to Ski Vorlage, located near the picturesque village of Wakefield, Quebec, in the Gatineau Hills. It was so beautiful and white, not the biggest ski place but perfect for me at that time. I had missed all the winter sports, but at the same time, I was so nervous.

The first time going down, I fell down, and I couldn't get up. Melissa helped me up, and I kind of slipped down the hill on my butt. At the bottom, I knew I was done, and I started slowly skiing toward the lodge—it was going to be a long day of pouting!

On my way back, Melissa and Tripp, Melissa's boyfriend at the time (fiancé now), kept insisting I try it one more time, and we kept arguing back and forth. He is one persistent man because I reluctantly followed them back to the top of the slopes. And I had the best time! I would fly down the moderate slope, faster than I should and out of control, and when my leg gave out, Tripp would come to help me get up again. That was the most fun I had in a long time.

On my last descent before lunch, I went down in a skier's crouch, pretending I was racing, and did my breaking at the bottom, making a snow shower. I loved it, then I fell, full of laughter and pure joy. At the bottom of the slope, I was sitting in the snow with the biggest smile like a little kid.

This woman, who had previously had to fetch my ski, stopped beside me and said, "You know you don't have to go so fast if you can't do it. You should slow down and ski with more control."

My smile changed to anger. I took a deep breath and said as calmly as I could, "I have MS, and this is probably the last time I will ever ski," and she skied away toward the ski lift.

After lunch, I went back with my son, Tristan, but my leg was no longer half working. It had died on me. I thought to myself, *I should never have gone in to have lunch*!

Honestly, I could go on and on about each physical ability that I've lost, but nothing could have prepared me for my mental abilities spiraling down. I felt like I was falling off a cliff. It started when Melissa was a teenager in high school and lasted into her adulthood! When she would speak to me, I would be so slow to respond, and she would get so angry and frustrated with me.

"Mom, why are you always ignoring me? You never answer me! I don't get that!"

Melissa was always very good at expressing herself.

"I was still thinking about the answer, and I was about to answer, but you didn't give me time to respond," I blurted back, and she would walk away, frustrated.

"Wait! It's my MS. It's not that I don't want to answer you. It's because it takes me a long time to process the information."

It would leave both of us so frustrated.

Many times, I would go to my room and cry about it. I couldn't even have a discussion with my own daughter, and she felt like I didn't listen to her.

In reality, I was dealing with brain fog! *Big time*! I was always exhausted and super tired. It didn't help that I couldn't sleep. The worst part was that I couldn't process what people were telling me. By the time I would think about the answer, they would be talking about something else. And I couldn't remember anything.

John and I would constantly argue about work. John would say, "I told you about that!" And I would get angry about it because I thought he didn't tell me. We would also argue about our children when we disagreed about whether they should go out or not. It became so difficult to think and process information that I didn't express myself. I also felt like I should avoid stress; therefore, I avoided confrontations. I avoided conversations. I became a silent partner in the family, living in my head with my own thoughts.

In the end of August 2019, it became so bad that it affected my work. I would come home from the office, eat lunch, and collapse on the couch for the rest of the afternoon. That was when I made the most important decision concerning my disease. *I changed my diet*!

Apart from turning my life to God and his help, the best thing that improved my health and well-being was a new diet. It happened when I was interested in a new device called PoNS that people would put on their tongue while they exercised. It would send electrical impulses to your brain and help you walk better and easier. The device had just been approved in Canada, and I called a doctor in Montreal, Canada, to see if I could participate in the program.

He informed me that without Canadian health insurance, it could cost me something like thirty thousand dollars, but while waiting its approval in the US, I should follow the diet that his neurological clinic advised with the program. It was called The Wahls Protocol. He emailed me the information about it, but I ignored it.

Who wants to give up eating cheese and bread and sugar? I'm not allergic to those things! I thought.

However, on one of those afternoons I was lying on the couch instead of working, I was desperate. I started doing some research on this diet on YouTube and on the doctor. Dr. Wahls was a medical doctor who ended up in a wheelchair because of MS and did her own research on what foods would heal you, and now she could walk and bike.

What did I have to lose?

The more I researched it, the more I realized that this was the third time that someone told me about this diet.

God, I will try it for two or three months, but if it doesn't work, I will go back to my normal diet, but maybe this is your answer to help me.

So I got on Amazon, and within two days, I was in possession of Dr. Wahls's diet book and her recipe book. According to her, all auto-immune diseases are caused by inflammation combined with missing important nutrients to fight the disease. The diet simply eliminates gluten, sugars, and dairy products because those can all cause inflammation! Eliminating all that good food sounded so crazy to me! No wonder it took me to be stuck on the couch to even want to try it. Fortunately, her diet offers three levels depending on whether you want to go very restrictive or a little less. In addition to avoiding all foods causing inflammation, every day, you basically eat a plate of greens, a plate of sulfur foods, as she calls it, such as onions and cabbage, and a plate of colorful vegetables and fruits, in addition to good proteins and fat. I decided to try the second level.

After three days of trying the second level, I didn't see much difference, but I kept a journal as she suggested, and I realized that I felt worse after I ate. I believe that my body was so bad off that it wasn't digesting food properly! I then decided to try the third and hardest level, which you only eat twice a day to allow your body to digest and heal. That made sense to me, but ouch, that was going to be difficult! To my amazement, after five days on the third level, my brain fog was gone. I could communicate with people and process information.

John said, "Wow, you remember what I tell you!"

One afternoon, after eating lunch, I was walking in the parking lot at work.

Oh my god! Thank you! Instead of lying on the couch, I'm walking.

I was so excited that I called my sister Melanie in Canada and told her all about the diet and how I felt good. I even placed an order on Amazon and had the same books delivered to her. She was also dealing with chronic inflammatory demyelinating polyneuropathy (CIPD), which is similar to MS except the peripheral nerves are affected as opposed to the brain.

To this day, I feel normal. No more brain fog! I can talk with people and work, and I no longer get MS tiredness or fatigue anymore. I can now fully enjoy spending time with people I love, including spending time with friends! I hope I never take that for granted again.

One of the greatest joys to me is to simply talk with my family: Melissa, Tristan, John, Peggy, and my Canadian family! I have missed that so much!

The best moment that will always keep a special place in my heart occurred a few months ago with my daughter, Melissa. I was able to drive to Raleigh, North Carolina, a one-and-a-half-hour drive with my new car hand controls, go out to eat, and see a play with her. Then I spent the night at her apartment, and the next day, as I was driving home, I couldn't help but smile. I could spend time with my daughter and hold a conversation with her! It was so nice, so amazing to me. I had gotten back what I had lost! What a gift!

CHAPTER 11

Still My Way or the Highway

THE SUMMER OF 2021, BEFORE I MET Annie Ruth and she told me to write this book, I felt great, and I believed that walking more normally again was the last piece of the puzzle in dealing with my MS.

As I previously mentioned, I felt great mentally, and I was now sleeping at night. I believed that I needed to find a good physical therapist who could help me use the new technology with stim, electrical current, to speed up the recovery of weak muscles. Professional athletes were now using that technology to speed up their recovery after they sustained injuries. I decided to pray for it. Honestly, with COVID-19, we had stopped going to church, and I was quite happy with my quiet life at home, not reading the Bible much or praying, but nonetheless, I decided to pray about it.

"God, help me find a physical therapist who can help me work out with a stim machine or help me to simply find the right physical therapist!"

On one of those weekends of that summer, we went to the beach, and Melissa brought her two friends, Sim and Liz, two of her best friends I really liked. One evening after dinner, I was sitting beside Liz who had previously told me that she was finishing a doctorate in physical therapy. I started explaining to her what I wanted to try, physical therapy combined with stim.

"Are you familiar with that?" I asked.

"No, I'm not, but it sounds interesting! I can try to find out more about it for you. Right now, I'm involved with a new program called MSFit, a program to help people with MS with exercise and physical therapy. If you're interested, I can give your name to my teacher who is also the administrator of this new program."

"I'm very interested, but it's a two-and-a-half-hour drive from Goldsboro to Winston Salem."

"I think because of COVID-19, they will also provide online therapy sessions!"

"I would love that! You can sign me up!"

"Okay, it starts in the fall semester, and I will text you when it starts. I'll get your phone number from Melissa."

A couple months later in the fall, Liz contacted me, and I scheduled an online physical therapy (PT) session with Dr. LaVerene Garner. I was so nervous because I was to do PT in front of Dr. Garner and ten to twenty graduate students. If it helped them and helped me at the same time, I was thankful for that. Lava, as I called her, was great!

In a nutshell, I prayed a simple prayer one-and-a-half-years ago, and God answered my prayer with providing the best physical therapist for me. She has been helping me since then. For the first time since my soccer career ended, I have been following an exercise program, and I have loved every second of it.

When I wake up, my amazing husband brings me coffee at 6:00 a.m., and I sit on the floor and begin my gentle stretches while I drink my coffee. I cannot function without stretching because I have spasticity, which in layman terms is simply stiffness that makes it hard to bend my legs. Once I finish my coffee, I proceed to my floor exercises with the exercises that Lava has given me. I love it—once again, I'm on a training program! Then, throughout the day, I have to keep track of my steps to eventually come to a total of five thousand steps!

The first few weeks and months, I was all-in and pushing myself to the limit, and then I would crash and get stiffer. And I would have to stop and recover and start over. Then I would do the same thing with the exercises and push and push while doing them the wrong way!

Lava kept me straight a few times and said, "Fab, sit down and listen to me if you want me to keep helping you! I used to work with the Marines, and like you, they pushed and pushed to their limits, but once they listened to me, they began to get better. I want you to walk a little at a time all day long and gradually increase your steps each week! Not walking and exercising so hard and crashing!"

Well, it did not take me long until I was walking my five thousand steps, but we discovered that I was doing all the exercises and walking incorrectly. I was walking mainly using my left leg, swinging my arm to the left, twisting my body in a weird way, and walking without using my abs. I was also doing the same thing with my strengthening exercises.

For example, I was doing squats with only my left leg. My abs would be so sore simply by doing breathing exercises done the right way. My abs, hip flexors, and right leg were so weak that it was like starting over. When I started doing my ab breathing exercises, I was doing only two thousand steps a day; thankfully, I am back to three thousand five hundred and gradually getting stronger and increasing my steps. I have no doubt that I will continue to slowly improve and slowly get stronger because nerves take longer than muscles to heal.

For example, the first time I was able to do two repetitions of my ab exercise, Lava got all excited.

"That's great! Two reps!"

That was when I realized it was going to be a long, long process! *But I was wrong about the last piece of the puzzle!*

I was so wrong thinking that my walking was the last piece of the puzzle—God had something else in mind. He was tired of my not following him and wanting to do it my way and really only praying every four years when I needed him. *He wanted all of me! All the time! Every second!* With this new PT, I was especially back to my old habits—I was training hard and accomplishing some great progress on my own effort. *But God wanted me to include him in my life!*

I believe that the bugle that Annie Ruth and Peggy heard was most likely to get me to write a book for God's glory and completely turn my life back to Jesus. Often, I am so stubborn and stuck in my ways that God has to knock me on the head literally! The last few months have been quite an adventure!

Where to begin?

First, you have to know that with COVID-19, I was quite happy living quietly at home, no one or nothing bothering me. I soon realized that I could no longer walk with shoes; it was very easy walking five thousand steps with no shoes! Lava told me that with a person who has MS, walking with shoes can be like walking with weights attached to your ankles.

Second, I realized that, mentally, I could not handle people anymore. For instance, the first time that I went to PNC Arena to watch the Carolina Hurricanes' hockey game, I could not handle it. With all the people walking around me, I couldn't walk because I thought they were going to hit me. My brain could not handle all that noise and so many people talking around me. I felt like I was going crazy—my brain was overloaded with echo. I just wanted to go home. I realized that I had to start getting out more and gradually start living a normal life again, which brought me to my other problem.

My other problem, my biggest problem, was that I wanted to go in public, but I didn't want anyone to see that I could no longer walk without using my poles. And also walking with poles was not pretty, especially when I worried on how it looked. I started texting my friend Kim Henderson and started going out with her once a month.

Every time I went out with her, I worried so much that she would see me not be able to walk that it would get worse and worse. Sometimes, I would walk normally in the house in the morning, but by the time I had to leave, I could hardly move. Stress was affecting my walking big time!

But it really became obvious that I had a huge problem in my last PT session in person. My husband and I drove to Winston Salem, North Carolina, to meet Lava. As I was getting ready in the hotel room, I started stressing so much that my blood pressure and heartbeat spiked up past normal readings.

As we drove there and as we waited for the appointment once there, I became more and more anxious. When she finally sat me on the table, I just started venting.

"I don't know what's wrong with me, but I make myself so nervous that it affects my walking. Then I worry so much that I won't be able to do the exercises because I get worse and worse with worry!

And I do the same when I go out with friends—I don't like for people to see me not able to walk."

"Fab, I'm a physical therapist, not a psychiatrist. I really believe that you should get help. I know of a good one here in Winston Salem, but you might want to get one close to where you live."

"Okay, let me see if I can find one in my hometown."

The rest of the session went better and better as I started relaxing.

On the drive back, I told John, "I was thinking of calling Viv so she can help me with my anxiety problem. What do you think?"

Vivienne was my sister-in-law. We had just visited them in Toronto, Canada, and had a great visit. I felt very comfortable with her.

"That's a great idea! I think that she could really help you!"

A couple days later, I was talking on the phone with Viv, and she was a great listener.

"Viv, I have some issues! This is so hard—I've always been the fastest and strongest, and now I have to depend on other people. Before COVID-19, I was able to hide that walking was very difficult, but I could still walk from A to B and pretend that everything was normal! If I needed to rest or stop, I would pretend to have to look at my phone or talk to someone. I was faking it big time! Now I have to use my poles, and I can't hide when walking like a cripple! I start stressing, knowing people are watching me, then stress affects my walking, making it more strenuous. And on and on it goes! It's a cataclysmic cycle for me! People constantly offer to help me, and it is so hard to accept."

It felt so good to actually talk about it for a third time, but in the end, she couldn't help me because she was only licensed to work in Ontario, Canada. I sure didn't want her to lose her license.

As we were ending the conversation, I strongly felt that I hadn't even thought of giving this problem to God, and so I told her, "I didn't even pray to God about this. I will do that first, then if I still have issues, I will see a psychiatrist."

CHAPTER 12

God's Way, Halfway

On October 29, 2022, I sat down by myself, no, not by myself. It was just me and God. I had just finished reading *Walking Through Fire* by Vaneetha Rendell Risner a second time. Victoria, my son's girlfriend, had suggested that I read that book. It was about a woman who had polio, and she thought that I would be able to relate to her.

The first time, I read the book straight through out of curiosity! However, I was not ready to deal with all the common issues that we shared: being slower than others, walking in a strange way, pretending everything was okay when it was not, just to name a few. And I certainly didn't want to learn to praise God in the midst of my sufferings and hardships! For that reason, I set the book aside.

On that day, in the solitude of my home, I had recently finished reading the book a second time! I had taken the time to ponder and pray about my disease, realizing that I had to stop letting my MS affect my whole life in a negative way. Like her, I made a list of all the things that I lost because I had MS. And it was a long list! The hardest one was not to be able to share different activities with my loved ones, like hiking! Then, to deal with this, I wrote down three scriptures to deal with them:

- "Come to me, all who labor and are heavy laden, and I will give you rest. Take my yoke upon you and learn from me; for I am gentle and lowly in heart, and *you will find rest* for your souls. For my yoke is easy, and *my burden is light*" (Matthew 11:28–30; italics mine).

- "Can any one of you by worrying add a single hour to your life?…Therefore *do not worry* about tomorrow, for tomorrow will worry about itself. Each day has enough trouble of its own" (Matthew 6:24–34; italics mine).
- "Forget the former things; do not dwell on the past. See, *I am doing a new thing*" (Isaiah 43:18; italics mine).

The second thing to deal with was all my fears that came with MS. My main two fears on this list were not being able to hold my grandchildren in my arms safely in the future and becoming a burden on my loved ones. Those were weighing heavily on my heart! The two Bible quotes I chose were

- "So *do not fear, for I am with you*; do not be dismayed, for I am your God. I will strengthen you and help you; I will uphold you with my righteous right hand" (Isaiah 41:10; italics mine).
- "There is no fear in love, *but perfect love casts out fear*" (1 John 41:10; italics mine).

The last one was dealing with my anger. I thought I had dealt with a lot of anger many years ago, but I still had anger in my heart especially about my walking, and more often than not, I let my anger about my walking affect the rest of my day.

- "*Trust in the LORD with all your heart* and lean not on your own understanding; in all your ways submit to him, and he will make your paths straight" (Proverbs 3:5–7; italics mine).

To sum it up, my new mantra was based on Philippians 4:4–7 that says:

> *Rejoice* [emphasis mine] in the Lord always.
> I will say it again: Rejoice! Let your gentleness be
> evident to all. The Lord is near. Do not be anx-

ious about anything, but in every situation, by prayer and petition, with thanksgiving, present your requests to God.

Basically, from now on, I will not wait for my walking to be perfect to enjoy life.
Pray and cheer up!

CHAPTER 13

Stubborn, God Hits Me on the Head

Shortly after this, right before Thanksgiving, we were driving to Raleigh, North Carolina, and my husband said, "You must really feel like you have to meet her for you to want to drive all the way to Raleigh to see someone you don't know!"

"Yes! By the way, her name is Vaneetha—she has polio and has written and published a book. But I have no idea why I'm going. Blame that one on Victoria! She had told me that it would be great if we could both meet!"

I also explained to him that I had done a quick prayer after Victoria spoke to me.

"God, you know I don't like to meet new people, but I will if you really want me to. I will not worry about it unless Victoria sets it up."

Satisfied, I moved on with my life. I also told him that on September 17, 2022, I received a text from Victoria: "Hi, Fab! I've been talking with my friend about you meeting with her mom, Vaneetha. She really wants to meet with you and was wondering if November 20 would work?"

"How well do you know her?" I had asked her.

"I've been best friends with her daughter, and we went to school together, and our families are good friends! My parents even went to their wedding!"

And now we were on our way to her house in Raleigh!

Now, looking back at the meeting, I realize that I was under the impression that Vaneetha wanted to meet me while she thought that I wanted to meet her. At first, it was a little awkward, but it became easier as I explained to her that I was also writing a book. She gave me great advice on how to get it published. However, I learned so much just watching her interact with her family. It was okay to live normally with a handicap and not let it affect your family life as I watched her interact with her husband and daughter in her house and knowing that she also helped a lot of people with suffering. It was eye opening for me! A moment in life that has helped me a lot in dealing with MS!

With all the godly events occurring in my past in a sporadic way, especially when I cried out to him in my suffering, and the bugle that got me to meet Annie Ruth who also told me that God wanted me to write a book and then having a meeting set up for me to meet an author, I was still bucking. It had been over a year since I started writing my book, and even after the meeting with Vaneetha, who had told me to write my book, I was still skipping more weekends and not writing.

I was a math brain. Why do I have to write a book? Maybe next weekend! I thought *until God knocked me on the head! Literally!*

It all started right before Thanksgiving; I was feeling pretty good. I always felt good when my walking and exercises were increasing at a good pace. Life was great. Thanksgiving was almost here, and I looked forward to seeing the whole family!

Then, all of sudden, as I was putting my walking poles in the back of the car, I started falling backward and landed on my tailbone on the concrete driveway. And I yelled loudly "Ouch!" as I laid there motionless and in pain. No one was around, and I was in no rush to move. Slowly, I sat up while pondering what had happened.

What the heck happened? I've been feeling great. I have no weaknesses at the moment, and I'm not tired! I don't understand.

I could not figure this one out.

Approximately one week later, I was starting to feel better. This time, I had to push myself a little harder to get ready for work and finally made it to the car.

Driving to work, I told myself, *I better be careful when I get there—I can't afford to fall again!*

Once inside our office building, I was fully aware that I was physically spent, and I thought that I would be wise to sit on the kitchen floor and rest. Instead, I told myself, *I can make it to my desk. I'm only a few steps away!*

As I was having those thoughts, I felt my body falling with my backpack holding my computer on my back.

Oh no! I cannot fall on my computer; I cannot lose all my files before I save them.

Midway to the floor, I grabbed the refrigerator handle, and instead of keeping me from falling, I dragged the fridge a short distance with me. I landed on my side with a loud yell and bang, while the bag went flying three feet from me! This time, I lay there a lot longer than the previous week, moaning in pain. It was my rib again! I knew all about those! Fortunately, it wasn't as bad as the last time that I had fallen on my rib. Unfortunately, it meant that I had to walk with my poles for a while and put my training schedule on hold. The good news was that the computer was intact and still functioning!

Two falls was not enough to get my full attention. Just as God had spoken to me three times in the past, on a Friday, December 9, 2022, I fell a third time, on my head, and hard!

All day that Friday, we were all at the office because it was raining. The work crews could not work in the rain because they needed to protect the expensive surveying instruments, so everyone got busy catching up on office work and repairs or car maintenance.

At the end of the day, only Tristan and I were left finishing our computer work. All day, I had been very careful moving around and always using my poles to make sure that my tailbone and rib were fully healed before attempting to walk without assistance!

At the end of the day, I got up to go use the bathroom. I was thinking about what we were going to do that weekend, and on the way, I stopped at Tristan's office's doorway to also discuss his weekend plans. Then I proceeded to the bathroom, still pondering everything, then suddenly, I had foot drop. My foot dragged on the floor, and I felt myself falling headfirst toward the wall.

Bang was followed by "*Owwww!*"

I lay there, lamenting in pain, while Tristan kept repeating, "Do I need to take you to the hospital? Oh my gosh! Your forehead—it's so big! Do I need to take you to the hospital?"

I slowly sat up, feeling my head was going to explode.

"I tell you what. I will let you drive me home and help me to the couch. You can get me some ibuprofen and ice for the swelling, and I will follow a concussion protocol, and then if it gets worse, you can drive me to the hospital" I bravely assured him but not feeling so sure myself.

"Okay, but you cannot watch TV or look at your phone either for a while!" he warned.

"That's fine! I will just lay there with my eyes closed and rest while I ice my head. But that was so stupid. I was using my poles all day long, and then I just forgot to use them to go to the bathroom. That was so stupid!"

Later at home, I was lying on the couch by myself, and I had just finished icing again. John and Tristan were resting in their bedrooms after they realized I was going to be okay and the lump on my forehead had gone down. It had been a hard week at work. I had been lying there with no TV and no phone, and I realized that we are so addicted to those things and to noise.

In the silence, at first, I was bored and craving to check my phone. Then I started wondering what happened and what was going on. Honestly, I felt like Job and pondered, *Does God want me to include him more? I have been neglecting him lately and not writing my book.*

So, finally, in the silence, I prayed, "*God, I don't know what to do about the falling, but you got my full attention. What do I have to do about this? Do I have to submit more? I don't know what to do. Tell me.*"

Realizing that I didn't have a concussion, I decided to keep all the electronics off and continue reading my book *Be Anxious for Nothing* by Joyce Meyers. I had decided to read it earlier to help me deal with my anxiety about not walking perfectly in front of other people and also to cast all my cares or problems on God.

In total silence and my total submission, in total humility instead of pride, in total dependence instead of independence, God spoke to me as I read that book. Joyce Meyers explained how King Jehoshaphat and the people of Judah faced their overpowering enemies and how we can apply it to our own lives (page 69):

> "For we have no power to face this vast army
> that is attacking us. We do not know what to do,
> but our eyes are upon you." (2 Chronicles 20:12)

I was amazed that it was exactly what I had prayed for! So I prayed it again but putting my situation in the verse: "For I have no power to face these falls that are attacking me. I don't know what to do, but my eyes are upon you."

Then Joyce Meyers went on to say that once we have (1) acknowledged that we have no power to save ourselves, (2) admitted that we do not know what to do about our situation, and (3) turned our eyes upon the Lord, placing our faith and trust in him to deliver us, then and only then you can take the next step:

> "This is what the Lord says to you: Do
> not be afraid or discouraged because of this vast
> army [these falls]. For the battle is not yours but
> God's." (2 Chronicles 20:15)

And then to:

> "Take up your positions; stand firm and
> see the deliverance the Lord will give you…" (2
> Chronicles 20:17)

Once again, God had to get my attention three times, including falling on my head, for me to completely depend on him. I started to cast all my care upon him, to pray and be thankful whether I walked two steps, two thousand steps, or five thousand steps. That was not my problem but his problem. Moreover, if he wanted me to write a book, I would. If he wanted me to publish it, that was also his problem, not mine. Maybe the book was only for my healing. We shall see.

For the next three months, I wrote more than I had in over a year!

CHAPTER 14

Deeper, All the Way

THREE MONTHS LATER, THINGS WERE GREAT. SPIRITUALLY and mentally, I was casting everything to God and learning to enjoy every day, knowing that God was in control. Even, physically, my walking was improving slowly.

Earlier in the month, I even enjoyed watching the Carolina Hurricanes live. I had no problems socializing and dealing with the loud noises. I actually enjoyed it! I was in a good place. And I had prayed that if God wanted anything different from me or wanted to use me, I was available. I was happy to keep things simple and as is, but I sure didn't want to oppose him anymore.

It was a beautiful, sunny Saturday in late March, and I had just finished my morning walk when Nancy, my neighbor, texted me: "U busy."

"I'm sitting on my front porch, enjoying the weather, if you want to join me," I replied, thinking it would be nicer to catch up in the sunshine than to be inside my house. I don't think that we had spoken in over a year. Chris, her husband, was a preacher, and he had just started a new church, which kept both of them very busy doing the Lord's work.

"Awesome," she texted back, and two minutes later, she joined me on the porch. We talked for an hour or two as if we had been talking to each other every day. It was a very deep conversation. She told me that Chris had just been diagnosed with myasthenia gravis (MG), an autoimmune disease similar to MS that causes a breakdown in the normal communication between nerves and muscles.

Some of the symptoms include weakness of arm or leg muscles, double vision, drooping eyelids, and difficulties with speech, chewing, swallowing, and breathing.[1]

We discussed how they were dealing with it, and I shared how I was dealing with my MS. I was glad that I could listen to her and tell her how I dealt with it. In the end, I shared with her that I was writing a book and that it had started with my mother-in-law hearing a bugle and my watching the video about the Bible passage "Speak, Lord, for your servant is listening" (1 Samuel 3:9).

And that I had specifically prayed, "Lord, speak to me through Annie Ruth tomorrow." And that the next morning, she had told me that God had spoken a word for her to tell me to write a book. And no, I was not a writer but a math person—I didn't understand, but who was I to argue with God? I was done with that, but be careful what you pray for.

Four days later, Nancy, my neighbor, rang my doorbell for a second time that week. She was almost out of breath when she asked me if I had a certain channel. She explained to me that her son was doing his internship in Texas, and they were going to cover it on TV. After looking for the channel without success, she rushed out the door to drive to her other son's house, Brian's, to videotape it. Shortly after, she reappeared at my door again, all excited to show me the video, and I was very glad to share her excitement.

After, I asked her how her church was doing and how many people were attending. I was asking because I had never found a small group like we used to have once a week. Throughout most of my children's middle and high school, we had a small prayer group of about five to eight people to pray for our children, their teachers, and our husbands. I missed that—I never felt that I fitted in any big church.

When she told me the number, I thought, *Nah, that's too big.*

Then she explained that they met on Wednesday night, and again I thought, *Too big.*

Then she got all excited.

"Oh! We have a women's Bible study starting tomorrow! And oh! It starts with your quote: '*Speak, Lord, your servant is listening*' [1

Samuel 3:9], the same quote that you mentioned that was the reason you were writing a book. I will be right back!"

And she ran out the house and came right back, out of breath, holding a small book. She opened it to show me that she signed it and also to show me the first page with the words: "Speak, Lord, for your servant is listening" (1 Samuel 3:9).

"How many people go to it?" I asked, thinking, *I don't want to join a big group.*

"Eight, maybe ten."

Crap! That's a perfect size. What's my excuse? I was thinking.

"Tell you what—I will pray about it and let you know tomorrow morning."

After she left and we finished eating supper, I found myself alone, sitting on the floor in my den, and opened the book that she had just given me called *Whisper* written by Mark Batterson. I love to read, and I opened the book to the prologue joyfully, and there it was on the first page: "Speak, Lord, for your servant is listening" (1 Samuel 3:9).

The prologue summarized the book's message about how to hear God as he speaks to us. Mark Batterson asked, "Would you be willing to pray a bold prayer at the beginning of this book?" Then he offers a seven-word prayer that can change a person's life: "Speak, Lord, for your servant is listening" (1 Samuel 3:9).

Then, in chapter 1, he talks about how he challenged his church to pray the bravest prayer they could pray. By bravest prayer, he means "the prayer that you can barely believe God for because it seems impossible and that it's often the prayer you've prayed a hundred times that hasn't been answered."

Then my husband, John, walked in and asked, "Am I disturbing you? I can leave."

"No, you're not. I was just finished."

Then we just watched TV and had a normal night together, quiet and relaxing, enjoying each other's presence, the book out of my mind.

The next morning, my wonderful husband brought my coffee, then I played scrabble on my phone, and he watched the news, a very normal routine for us. Then he left for work, and I started my floor exercises while listening to Christian music.

As I was lying on my back and starting with my leg exercises with a rubber band, I began to feel overwhelmed with the day ahead of me. I had to drive my mother-in-law around on that day because her car was getting fixed. And if I decided to go to the women's Bible study, that would be more sitting. To be at peace with it, I started praying while still exercising.

"Please, Lord, just help me walk today after driving so much. You know how my right leg gets really tight after driving and sitting a lot. Please, I just want to be able to get around easily with my poles."

That was when I heard, "*That is not bold enough.*"

It was a whisper in my spirit, loud and clear, like it was described in the book the previous night. I stopped exercising.

God, do you want me to pray to walk normally?

I took a breath.

Without poles?

I took another breath.

With my family members?

Another breath.

And not be left behind when they're walking somewhere?

Then I heard the next song: "…step by step…"

Oh, God! I want to walk with my family members, with people I love, without poles! Is that bold enough? I want to walk normally with them and enjoy them. Is that bold enough?

At this point, I was weeping, and tears were flowing down my face.

The next song was on: "…I'm your cornerstone…"

I kept crying joyfully.

Then I heard more singing: "…Jesus died for you…"

Tears were still rolling down my face when I texted Nancy: "I will go tonight. Just tell me what time you will pick me up."

And for good measure, I prayed my boldest prayer: "Lord, help me walk normally, without poles with my family members!"

And I checked the date on my phone: 3/30/23.

After an emotional day, thinking about my morning's boldest prayer and enjoying spending time with my mother-in-law, getting my hair trimmed and eating lunch together, I was tired by the time Nancy picked me up in the evening. And of course, my walking was difficult; my right leg was tight and weak.

I honestly told Nancy, "I'm not sure why I'm going, and I'm missing my hockey game."

I repeated it again, and I was feeling tired. Pouting might better to describe how I reacted to being dragged out of my comfort zone!

When we arrived there, I took three or four steps and stopped. Again, I took another three or four steps and stopped. Nancy was holding the door open. It felt like an eternity for me to just get through the door while they waited on me.

Inside, I spotted Savannah, my massage therapist, who had been helping me with my leg stiffness for about a year.

At least, I knew someone! I thought as she ended up sitting beside me.

As I was sitting there, I noticed the sheet that was on the table in front of me. It listed the budget and the calendar of activities coming up. I wondered if I had to sit through the budget meeting before we started the Bible study.

Okay, I need to change my attitude. Lord, you want me here—I'm all yours. Fill me with your Holy Spirit.

Shortly after that moment, Nancy came back and sat beside me on the vacant chair. She had disappeared at the beginning and had left me alone to converse with the group of women. She leaned over and whispered in my ear, "I know why you're here!"

Wondering what she meant, I continued to listen to the women discussing the book *Whisper.*

After the budget meeting and our women's Bible study, Nancy and another woman were putting up the food in the kitchen while I waited and stretched in the other room. Sure enough, they both came out, and Nancy said, "Fab, I want you to meet Christie. She was just diagnosed with MS today!" For a minute, I was speechless.

God, forgive me. Here I am, use me to help her if she needs it.

Now I knew why she had been missing for most of the meeting—she was probably crying in another room or in the bathroom.

I got up and walked toward her and gave her a big hug.

"I'm so sorry," I said, feeling emotional and knowing all the difficulties she would be dealing with. I could empathize.

We talked for almost two hours after everyone had left. I think that day, I made a new friend!

Driving home with Nancy, I let everything out.

"I don't understand," I said as I explained to Nancy all the godly moments that had been occurring. "Why me? I'm just happy doing my own thing, a simple life. What does God want from me?" I was so emotionally spent!

Nancy replied, "Fab, you're like Moses! Stop fighting it! God will equip you with everything you need to do his will."

Like Moses, I was full of excuses. When God told Moses that he was sending him to Pharaoh to bring the Israelites out of Egypt, Moses responded with several excuses:

1. Who am I?
2. What if they don't believe me or listen to me?
3. Lord, I am not eloquent enough.
4. Lord, please send someone else.

And that was when the Lord's anger burned (Exodus 4:1–15). And here I was doing the same thing.

I arrived home late and collapsed in bed. It took me two days to fully recover, not physically but emotionally and spiritually. I was so happy with my simple life, but God wanted more from me, so much more. That was so clear to me, but it was hard to accept and take the next step and step out of my comfort zone!

Happiness

LOOKING BACK ON MY LIFE, I HAVE been so blessed! I had awesome parents, great brother, and sisters. Then I lived my dreams and played soccer with the best players and was coached by the best while making friends for life. I am married and loved by the best husband with two great children. We also live in the freest and richest country in the world! Yet along the way, I often had it so wrong!

I never enjoyed where I was in life! I could be playing soccer in China, Holland, or anywhere. Instead of being upset about how I played, angry at a coach, or worried about my future career, did I enjoy the present? Did I get down on my knees and say "*Thank you, God*"? Did I just have fun doing what I love and fully appreciate it? I'm afraid not.

What about my children? It was always going to be better when I was able to walk better, have more money, or feel less tired. Do children care if you are not running or walking like you used to? *Thank you, God, for my awesome children*! Enjoy the moment; you will never have young children again!

What about criticizing my husband when he walks on my kitchen floor with his muddy shoes? Why not be thankful for him to still be beside me, supporting me and loving me! My husband will carry my surfboard for fifteen minutes to the beach and patiently wait until I walk to the edge of the ocean with my poles. Then he walks back to put my poles on top of our towels and walks back and pushes me in the deeper water just so I can float in the ocean. *Thank you, God, for such a great man*!

I was eight years old when I told my mom I was going to be in the Olympics. I believed that it was going to happen, but was I thankful that I was blessed with such athletic talent? Didn't God say that I was wonderfully made (Psalms 139:13–14)? Did I stop and really thank him for who he made me to be and for the dreams he gave me? I'm afraid that I did not. It became all about me, myself, and I. *Forgive me, Lord!*

I have been so selfish and stubborn. I am just realizing more fully that God has been pursuing me. It is overwhelming! Is God pursuing you? It took miracles and a bugle, and then he knocked me on the head. And I am just realizing that perhaps God didn't want to heal just my walking and my physical disabilities. And I was getting angry at the videos that described how 1 Peter 2:24 was talking about healing spiritually! And when Annie Ruth's son asked me what to pray about and I said "my walking!" then he responded "spiritual or physical?" and I was angry. Now I realized I needed to heal completely: emotionally, spiritually, and also physically. Now I try to live like God wants me to live.

God tells me to forget the former things, to not dwell on the past (Isaiah 43:18), to not worry about tomorrow (Matthew 6:34), and to pray for my daily bread (Matthew 6:11). It sounds too simple. Learn from the past but don't dwell on it. Plan for the future but don't stress about it and enjoy the present in its fullness.

Second, cast all your anxiety (your cares) on God because he cares for you (1 Peter 5:7). Again, it sounds too simple. Now when I start worrying, I give it all to God, and when I do that, it is no longer my problem. God is better-equipped than me to handle the problems.

Third, my son, Tristan, always tells me "Mom, it's okay to ask for help" when he sees me struggling with my disease. Honestly, asking for assistance is still one of the most challenging things for me to do. I am too proudful; I want to be independent and do it my way. Do you humble yourself and ask God for help? Every time I have been at my lowest point and cried out to God, my King, he has heard my voice (Psalms 5:2–3). Do you ask others for help? It is all right for my family and friends to carry my things or for strangers to open the door for me. Yet it is still difficult for me to let them. I am trying to humble myself, smile, and thank them when they help me (Matthew 23:12). This one is still a work in progress.

Fourth, love others. Ooh! That sounds too simple, but this is the hardest. Loving others when they are difficult to love is not easy. Loving includes forgiving, but do you forgive people who have hurt you? Good question. I know Jesus has forgiven me, and I know if I forgive someone, it doesn't mean what they have done is right, but it allows me to let go of it. And when I carry that burden, it hurts me, it hurts my health, so I try to forgive.

Fifth, I now try to obey God by doing everything for the Lord cheerfully because a cheerful heart is good medicine, but a crushed spirit dries up the bones (Proverb 17:22). Losing so much to a disease makes you enjoy menial tasks. Now I am so thankful when I can walk down the street, I sing when I can sweep the floor, and I smile when I can help someone. I want everything I do done for the glory of God (1 Corinthians 10:31). Do you take small things you do for granted? We all do. Appreciate your life because you are a very special person, and life is a gift!

Lastly, God, use me for your glory.

REFERENCES

Part 1

Chapter 1: Go Home or Go Broke

1. Gopack.com. "1987 Women's Soccer Schedule." https://gopack.com/sports/womens-soccer/schedule/1987.

2. Deuel, Scott. 1987. "Booters Open 1987 Season Impressively." *Technician*, vol. LXIX, no. 7 (September): 9. https://ocr.lib.ncsu.edu/ocr/te/technician-v69n7-1987-09-09/technician-v69n7-1987-09-09.pdf.

3. Deuel, Scott. 1987. "Booters Open 1987 Season Impressively." *Technician*, vol. LXIX, no. 7 (September): 10. https://ocr.lib.ncsu.edu/ocr/te/technician-v69n7-1987-09-09/technician-v69n7-1987-09-09.pdf.

7. Pacific Exchange Rate Service. https://fx.sauder.ubc.ca/etc/CADpages.pdf.

5. Society for American Soccer History. "USWNT Results: 1985–1989." https://www.ussoccerhistory.org/usnt-results/uswnt-results/uswnt-results-1985-1989/.

6. Wikipedia.com. "Canada Women's National Soccer Team Results, 1986–1988." https://en.wikipedia.org/wiki/Canada_women%27s_national_soccer_team_results.

4. Wikipedia.com "St. John's-Ravenscourt School." https://en.wikipedia.org/wiki/St._John%27s-Ravenscourt_School.

Chapter 2: Childhood Olympic Dream
4. 1976-RO-S-Montreal-Vol_1_III.pdf. "Official Ceremonies and the Olympic Flame," 286–287. https://stillmed.olympic.org/ Documents/Reports/Official%20Past%20 Games%20Reports/Summer/1976/ ENG/1976-RO-S-Montreal-Vol_1_III.pdf.
6. 1976-RO-S-Montreal-Vol_1_III.pdf. "The Torch Bearers and Escorts," 8. https:// stillmed.olympic.org/Documents/Reports/ Official%20Past%20Games%20Reports/ Summer/1976/ENG/1976-RO-S-Montre- al-Vol_1_III.pdf.
1. "Final 1987 Atlantic Coastal Conference Women's Soccer Summary." https://unc_ftp.sidearms- ports.com/custompages/Women's_Soccer/ 1987Stats.pdf.
3. Foisy, Paul. 2011. "The Montreal Olympics," updated by Tabitha Marshall, last edited March 31, 2016. https://www.thecanadi- anencyclopedia.ca/en/article/the-montreal- olympics.
2. Gopack.com. 2008. "NC State Women's Soccer History of Success." https://gopack.com/ news/2008/8/7/NC_State_Women_s_ Soccer_s_History_of_Success.
5. Olympics.com. "Montreal 1976: The Torch: Route Design and Detail." https://olympics. com/en/olympic-games/montreal-1976/ torch-relay.

Chapter 3: Cloud Nine and Then Some More
3. Drew, Jeff. 1990. "Booters Lose Nailbiter in Double Overtime." *Technician*, vol. 72, no. 34 (November): 5. https://d.lib.ncsu.

edu/collections/catalog/technician-v72n34-1990-11-12#?c=&m=&cv=4&xywh=-4648%2C0%2C18106%2C7100.

4. Drew, Jeff. 1990. "Booters Lose Nailbiter in Double Overtime." *Technician*, vol. 72, no. 34 (November): 8. https://d.lib.ncsu.edu/collections/catalog/technician-v72n34-1990-11-12#?c=&m=&cv=7&xywh=-6820%2C-1%2C18098%2C7098.

6. History Carolina Women Soccer. "The Greatest Game in Women's Soccer Lore," 35. http://catalog.e-digitaleditions.com/i/39090-2011-womens-soccer-yearbook/35.

5. Pekale, Zach. "Mia Hamm's College Career: North Carolina Highlights and Notable Moments." https://www.ncaa.com/news/soccer-women/article/2020-05-28/mia-hamms-college-career-north-carolina-highlights-and-notable-moments.

2. Ussoccer.com. 2019. "Jill Ellis—Farewell to the Winningest Coach in the US Soccer History." https://www.ussoccer.com/stories/2019/10/jill-ellis-farewell-to-the-winningest-coach-in-us-soccer-history.

1. Wikipedia.com. "NC State Wolfpack Women's Soccer: History: 1980s." https://en.wikipedia.org/wiki/NC_State_Wolfpack_women%27s_soccer#:~:text=1988%20was%20the%20Wolfpack's%20best,the%20team%20again%20enjoyed%20success.

Chapter 4: Big Plans, Big Crash

1. Wikipedia.com. "Anson Dorrance: National Team Coach." https://en.wikipedia.org/wiki/Anson_Dorrance.

2. Wikipedia.com. "Jill Ellis: Personal Life." https://en.wikipedia.org/wiki/Jill_Ellis.

3. Gopack.com. "1991 Women's Soccer Schedule." https://gopack.com/sports/womens-soccer/schedule/1991.

4. Drew, Jeff. 1991. "Women's Soccer Team Scores First Round NCAA Win." *Technician*, vol. LXXII, no. 34 (November): 3. https://ocr.lib.ncsu.edu/ocr/te/technician-v69n7-1987-09-09/technician-v69n7-1987-09-09.pdf.

5. Drew, Jeff. 1991. "Women's Booters Ousted by Tarheels." *Technician*, vol. LXXII, no. 37 (November): 3.

Part 2: Lost
Chapter 5: Diagnosis

2. Atkinson, Charles. 1994. "Greensboro Dynamo Fielding Women's Dawn of Women's Professional Soccer in America." *News & Record* (April, updated January 23, 2015). https://greensboro.com/greensboro-dynamo-fielding-womens-team-dawn-of-womens professional-soccer-in-america/article_5746c4d9-64df-50cc-95dc-9bad-c878aabb.html.

1. Wikipedia.com. "Montel Williams." https://en.wikipedia.org/wiki/Montel_Williams.

Chapter 7: God Heard Me

1. Alamy.com. 2002. Alamy Stock Photo. https://www.alamy.com/anne-graham-lotz-daughter-of-evangelist-billy-graham-addresses-the-crowd-during-the-just-give-me-jesus-revival-

saturday-april-27-2002-in-raleigh-nc-lotz-says-she-doesnt-have-the-gifts-that-made-her-father-the-20th-centurys-most-famous-evangelist-but-has-become-a-popular-speaker-among-evangelical-christians-in-america-and-around-the-world-ap-photonews-observer-sher-stoneman-image542992482.html.

Chapter 14: Deeper, All the Way
    1. Mayoclinic.org. "Myasthenia Gravis." https://www.mayoclinic.org/diseases-conditions/myasthenia-gravis/symptoms-causes/syc-20352036?utm_source=Google&utm_medium=abstract&utm_content=Myasthenia-gravis&utm_campaign=Knowledge-panel.

Chapter 5 through chapter 14
    Throughout chapters 5 through chapter 14, medical information, spiritual events, and time frame were reconstructed from my medical charts, personal journals, physical therapist programs, and appointments and also through emails and texts.

ABOUT THE AUTHOR

Fabienne Gareau Rudolph is a first-time author who resides in North Carolina with her husband, John, and enjoys spending time with her two grown children, Melissa and Tristan. She received her bachelor's degree from North Carolina State University where she also played soccer. Additionally, she played soccer for the Canadian Women's Soccer Team. She continues to learn how to live with her multiple sclerosis.

www.ingramcontent.com/pod-product-compliance
Lightning Source LLC
Chambersburg PA
CBHW022023150726
47990CB00002B/787